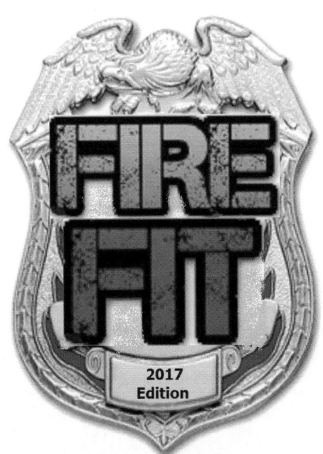

CHAD M. MCKINLEY
Trainer, Coach and Combatives Instructor

by Chad M. McKinley

Chad M. McKinley and M.A.C.
All Rights Reserved. No part of this publication may be reproduced in any form or by any means, including scanning, photocopying, or otherwise without prior written permission of the copyright holder. Copyright © 2016

Table of Contents

1. Introduction

2. SECTION I (The Knowledge Base)

3. Your Diet and Nutrition
4. Your Strategic Shake Diet
5. Your 100 Shake Recipes
6. Your Supplementation
7. Your Successful Sleep Strategy
8. Your balance and flexibility
9. Your Speed and Agility
10. Your Strength and Conditioning
11. Your Body-Weight Strategy: *Using a weight based upon your own body weight*
12. Your Cardio Training
13. Constructing your "Fitness Plan": *Becoming your own Trainer/Coach*

14. SECTION II (The Action Plan)

15. **Your Year Long Nutritional Plan :** Weight-Loss/Cut and Gain/Mass
16. **Your Year Long Cardio Plan :** Indoor and Outdoor
17. **Your Year Long Strength Plan :** Gym/Weights and No-Weight Option
18. **Your Year Long Conditioning and Drills Plan:** Speed, Agility, Defense
19. **Your Optional and Extra Workouts**
    - 19.1. TRACK Workout
    - 19.2. Bodyweight Workouts: *using your own body's full weight*
    - 19.3. MMA Drills: *Designed to enhance Combat performance*
    - 19.4. Years 2 and beyond Workouts

20. **Support Website , Printable Forms** and **Phone App**

21. **VIDEO SUPPORT:** New Training vids, Instructionals, How-To
22. **- Grocery List**
23. **Glossary**

1. Introduction

"The strategic application of all the newest in sports science combined with the best time proven techniques of the past"

After over two decades and hundreds of athletes and clients......I have taken and developed one of the top overall programs designed for achieving your goals and dreams.

I have accomplished this by combining an immense knowledge of your body's biomechanically efficient movement, the body's physiological capabilities, its weaknesses, its peak performance ....and its maximum required recovery.

I combined this with the latest in diet & nutrition and finish with a powerful program that will literally transform your body into a machine and transform YOU into your own coach / Trainer for the rest of your life.

When you start training on this program , you'll begin to develop an amazing ability to recover rapidly from intense workouts.

Fitness—like performance or competition—is not really a matter of **who can do more**, but in actuality is **who can do it more often**. It isn't about the one who can go the longest at an easy pace, but it is about the one who can perform a workout / compete and then shake it off and go at it again tomorrow ......who survives and thrives.

While I can't make you bullet-proof, I can make you injury-proof by giving your nervous system the ability to respond to sudden, overwhelming and forceful circumstances with ease and comfort. Then instruct you on the proper methods and techniques to fully recover and come back tomorrow for more.

For this reason a mandatory portion of the program approaches fitness from a "Self-Defense" or "Martial Arts" perspective.

Due to the extreme psychological stress experienced by Real-life " Warriors "…..……

Learning the same method that safely reabsorbs the **adrenal dump** of your "fight or flight" response mechanism is needed. You're of no help to yourself or others…… if you're always sick, burnt-out or exhausted all day from the high intensity of fitness training.

Imagine mastering all of these skills and then applying them to your current everyday life and stresses.

Accelerated recovery………in a life crisis and/or in your daily life…..will play a huge role into your achievement of your overall goals, overall happiness and daily peace-fo-mind.

My training methods will help you to recover your resting **heart rate and breathing rate……** *up to 6X faster than most highly conditioned athletes.*

And as anyone knows……The more relaxed your breathing and your body, the more steady and focused you will be.

Each "Phase" will incorporate and focus toward your chosen goal

- **High-Intensity Fat-Burning Circuits**: each workout in the program **can** be completed in less than 30 minutes and those 30 intense minutes will build and hone your desired skill-sets..... while also melting the fat faster than hours of your typical "cardio-style" exercises.

- **Specific Skills Development:** promotes *"neurological programming"*. Time will appear to slow down as you speed up, your fine motor skills will become more accurate, your gross motor skills more efficient and you will feel significantly less stress during performance and even more so in your daily life.

- **Tactical Applications**: each exercise has been put into practice for decades by my past athletes and clients and are carefully programmed to forge the highest level of specific conditioning while building and reinforcing all of your tactically relevant life and sport skill sets.

- **Injury-Proofing** and **Active Recovery**: specifically designed low-intensity mobility and agility exercises that are designed to accelerate your recovery from intense workouts, prevent you from overtraining and diminish the delayed muscle soreness that is typical of extreme exertion.....which translates to constant state of mission or performance readiness.

- **Functional Muscle**: All body movement requires moving muscle. And nothing builds ripped and usable muscle like having a huge array of exercises. That's the secret to the physique competitors, special ops guys and professional athletes.

They build **GO MUSCLE** ….. and ….. **SHOW MUSCLE**.

2. SECTION I (The Knowledge Base)

3. Your Diet and Nutrition

Diet and Nutrition Strategies

There are so many crazy diet fads out there that we have all lost count.
Yet while the diets don't seem to stay around long, people usually do seem get some mild results by following them.

People do technically lose weight.
So why is it that in the long run, none of these fad diets ever seems to work long-term?
Whether for weight-loss, gain or sports performance?

Most diets will work at least on a short term basis, but who wants to live their life half starving and depriving themselves of the foods they love?

With that said.....if you don't mind deprivation, then which diet is The right one right for you?

What is the final answer for healthy fat loss and muscle gain that you can and will stick with longterm?

Example:

In a single given year, Americans will consume roughly a billion dollars worth of bagels. This is just a single food!

Not to mention.... if your diet is asking you to give up a food you obviously love dearly, how long will you stick to it? I say.....Not very long!

This is why the low-carb food market has taken such a serious nose-dive.

At the complete other end of our dieting spectrum, a so-called **low-fat diet** causes a person's blood sugar levels to seriously fluctuate. This having a big impact on their moods and their appetites. This making them moody and hungry almost all the time.

Do you want to live like that?
Who wants to follow such an "extreme diet" that it deprives you of an entire macro-nutrient family, such as your carbohydrates and/or fats?

A more practical and beneficial diet would be one that allows for a balanced diet of proteins, carbs and fats, while still losing fat, being healthy and has you enjoying life. Diet is mainly about the old adage "*calories in and calories out*".

The main roadblock to dieting success stories is the finding of a diet you can stick with and that will work for you long term. If you absolutely hate to follow a specific diet regime, then you will not follow it in the long term.....taking you right back to the starting point.

We will lay out the specific diet principles for you that have been very successful for hundreds of my clients. Not only at improving appearance and self esteem, but also sports-performance.

If getting lean and in-shape while still enjoying your life are things that you are interested in, then I suggest that you continue to read on. This book might just change your life. This is no "dieting fad" or "exercise program" you have just purchased..... this is a Lifestyle upgrade!

This diet works because it is designed and custom-built by you to fit your schedule and your particular set of needs.
You are allowed to eat various varieties of foods without having to count every calorie you eat.

Dieting is very stressful already, without trying to calculate every single calorie you eat during a day.
Instead our Diet counts your "servings" of foods, which makes meal planning quite a bit easier. We recommend that you simply measure your food the first two weeks. This is to teach yourself what an actual "serving" really is and what it really looks like. Soon you will not need to measure everything, because you will already have learned to know how much of a certain food an actual "serving" is.

Why My Diet Strategy Works

The key to our Diet is that it MUST work for you and work well with your schedule. We ask you to give us 80% of the requested effort to follow the simple, delicious meal plans and you take 20% for yourself.

Meaning simply, that when Sunday night comes around and you want to go out and have dinner with your friends/family....Then do it. Ice cream on a Saturday Afternoon? Popcorn at the movies?
Do not fuss or stress about your diet!

All we ask is that the next day, you throw in a little extra cardio. Or simply take the dog or just yourself for an extra 10 minute walk ....and get right back on track with the nutrition portion of your program.

> We never want the meal plans to interfere with your daily life and plans.
>
> That is the entire premise of you learning to design them for yourself.

Another example:
On Saturday morning you want pancakes, eggs, bacon and hash browns.....have it! However, Do not think that you have to starve or not eat the rest of the day to make up for the larger breakfast meal. This is the last thing you want to do.

Your job is to get right back on track and get that second meal in as planned. Starving is definitely not our answer here. When you start starving yourself or forget to eat during the day, your body senses this and slows down your metabolic rate, because it thinks it does not have all the calories it will need to survive.

The body's goal is to survive! So when the body senses "starvation mode", it simply slows everything down to preserve energy stores.......also known as *fat tissue*.

This means that your 'fat burning' process is slowed down to preserve energy.
The goal of our diet is to keep the body running and therefore burning calories.
Every time we eat, our body has no choice but to burn calories just to digest the foods we have eaten. That is why we promote eating your meals frequently and spread out strategically throughout the day.
This literally promotes the constant burning of FAT.

By eating small, frequent meals, you also create a smaller insulin spike.
By eating more infrequently with higher calorie meals, you are causing a large insulin spike that can result in a blood glucose crash that also halts fat loss once again.
We want to keep insulin levels steady throughout the day.

By eating your smaller, more strategically placed meals....your bodies insulin levels will remain stable while you keep your metabolism revving, because your body is kind of like a furnace ; if you don't keep the coal in it, it will stop burning.

We also always include some kind of fat with our meals.
When you eat fat with any meal, especially one containing complex-carbohydrates, it reduces your bodies "gastric emptying" and allows your body to release insulin at a much slower and steady rate than by eating the carbohydrates alone.

The Keys To Burning Fat All Day Long

Calorie Control

· Even though you will probably end up eating more on this diet than on any diet you have ever done, the biggest factor in any good diet is "calories in versus calories out" with a myriad of versions of macro-nutrient manipulation.

· **Do not skip your meals:** Skipping meals will drastically reduce your blood sugar levels and make you crave sugary high calorie sweets later on.

· **Always Remember:** You are going to have to always be eating to LOSE or GAIN weight. Starving yourself may get you to lose a couple of quick pounds, but the repercussions of not eating and providing the body with the essential nutrients will lead you into an unhealthy lifestyle.
When you do not eat, the body senses there is no nutrition and its job now turns and becomes "Survive".

It will slow down your entire metabolic rate and begin to eat away at lean muscle tissue. This makes it extremely difficult to burn and lose body fat once you begin to eat again.

· **Be aware of the portion sizes of the food selections you make.**
One serving of spaghetti is a ½ cup AFTER its COOKED.
Most restaurants provide 4 or 5 servings per plate.

The key here is to eating until you are CONTENT and not until you are technically "FULL", nor the "Plate Empty".

Insulin Control

Insulin is referred to as your "storage hormone", because its job is to activate the transportation of nutrients (Such as carbs and fats) into your cells and to turn off the burning of the provided nutrients.

When you eat carbohydrates, blood glucose levels rise.....
which the body does not like.

In order to bring blood glucose levels back into the normal range, the pancreas secretes insulin. This signals cells to increase the uptake of glucose from the blood into them.
During this particular time, fat burning is completely shut-down.
Therefore what we want is to control insulin levels to keep fat burning elevated.

The Keys to doing this are:

· Eat five to eight small meals per day: a Large meal can create an enormous insulin spike, which will cause your body to store excess fat.
Small meals create a considerably smaller and more controlled insulin release, thus less fat storage and greater potential for fat loss.

· Never skip a meal: We don't care if meal one was at the local Chinese buffet and you ate until you had to unbuttoned your pants to breathe.
Do not skip your second, third and fourth meal! Keep your motor revving.

· Eat good fat with every meal, especially your carbohydrate meals.
As you will see, I prescribe Coconut Oil.

· Do not combine starchy-carbohydrates and high-protein in a meal, this elicits your highest insulin response. As an example, a cup of oatmeal has a moderate insulin response, however when you combine oatmeal with whey protein, you get a considerably greater response.

However, if you do happen to combine these, be sure to add a fat source.

You can already see the beginnings of your future meal planning taking shape here.
Carb meal, then Protein meal, Then Carb meal, then Protein
AND Carb ..... but WITH coconut oil (or another good fat source) added somewhere or somehow.

Acidity Control

What we are talking about here is the controlling the acidity of your meals.
Why is this important to us and how can this be accomplished?

· Your body pH level is slightly alkaline.
The normal range is 7.36 to 7.44.
To maintain your optimal health and achieve best results, you should attempt to keep your body in an alkaline state through your diet.
An imbalanced diet high in acidic foods will make your body quite acidic.
This might deplete the body of alkaline minerals such as sodium, potassium, magnesium, and calcium.
Thus making you more prone to chronic and degenerative diseases and potentially a disrupting of your overall nutrient absorption.

· Add fat to your meals. For example.... When you eat a meal of oatmeal and egg whites, you are consuming a very acidic meal. However when you add raisins and almonds into your oatmeal and add in some steamed vegetables, you are lowering the acidity level of that meal quite dramatically.
All of our Diet program meals keep this factor in mind.

· When you cannot add fat or vegetables to your meals, you can add two to five grams of L-Glutamine.
The glutamine will lower the overall acidity of your meal to keep you in a more alkaline state.
L-Glutamine can be purchased in pill form , is cheap and can be kept in your cars glove box.
Take two or three pills before going into a restaurant or wherever.

What are some Alkaline Foods?

Vegetables

Asparagus
Artichokes
Cabbage
Lettuce
Onion
Cauliflower
Radish
Watercress
Spinach
Green Beans
Celery
Cucumber
Broccoli

Fruits

Grapefruit
Banana
Lemon
Tomato
Watermelon
(neutral)

Nuts & Seed

Almonds
Pumpkin
Sunflower
Sesame
Flax

Fats & Oils

Avocado
Hemp
Flax
Olive
Coconut Oil
Borage

General Guidelines:

- Stick with salads, fresh veggies and healthy nuts and oils.
- Try to drink at minimum two to three liters of clean, pure water daily.

Hydration Control

You will need to drink plenty of water everyday.
Try drinking eight glasses (or 64 oz.) of water each day.
Your benefits of drinking throughout the day are to provide optimal hydration ,as well as, a feeling of "fullness" without any added calories.
While on a "Shake Diet".....This shouldnt be an issue.

Quality Control

· Choose fresh, wholesome foods over any pre-packaged or processed foods.
Packaged foods are usually loaded with preservatives, especially saturated fats and sodium, and are often high in amounts of added sugars, such as high fructose corn syrup.

It will amaze you how fast you can lose fat by just packing prepared meals from home rather than the purchasing of fast food or packaged foods.
You also will save a lot of money in the end.

· Eat one or two fruit servings and three to five vegetable servings each and everyday.
Fruits and vegetables are packed with fiber, antioxidants, vitamins and minerals.

One serving of vegetables equals one-half of a cup unless leafy.
One serving of leafy vegetables equals one cup.

Fruits and vegetables provide nutrient dense calories and healthy fiber.

Now that we have an understanding on the principles and keys to this diet, let's discuss nutrition.

What Is Nutrition?

Nutrition is the very science of our foods and nutrients and their actions within the human body.

This is including the ingestion, the digestion, the absorption, the transportation, the utilization and the excretion.

Nutrition has played a large role in your life, even before your birth and will continue to affect your life in large ways depending on the foods you choose to eat.

Food Selections:

People decide what they will eat and when they will eat it often based on social motives/objectives, rather than on their awareness of nutritional importance to their overall good health and performance.

The following are various behavioral and/or social motives for peoples food selections -

Body weight combined with personal image: Some people select certain foods and supplements that they feel and believe will improve their physical appearance and they also avoid foods they feel might be Detrimental or negative.
These decisions can be beneficial when based on sound nutrition and exercise information and science, but can be the Exact reverse if based on quick fixes and popular fads with no backing.

Availability, convenience and economy: People eat foods that are easily accessible, quick to prepare and within their financial means.
With today's daily stresses including work, children, finances, personal appearance....quick and easy selections can outweigh healthy nutrition selections at times.

Social interactions: Many people enjoy eating with their family and friends. Meals are social events and the sharing of food is part of our customs and hospitality.

Emotional comfort: Many people eat as a response to stress or an emotional stimulus. Eating in response to emotions and/or stress can lead to overeating and the following increased weight gain.

Personal preferences: People like certain foods based on flavor and taste.

Force of Habit: Certain foods are selected based on your individual habit. People will eat breakfast cereal every morning based solely on lifelong habit. Eating a familiar food and not having to make any real decisions can be easy and or less stressful and more comforting.

Ethnic heritage or tradition:
This is One of the strongest and biggest influences on food selections.
Different ethnic backgrounds tend to have staple foods that they use in their typical main dishes.

Positive and negative association: People seem to tend to like foods that were somehow related to a fun or happy moment in their life. On the other hand, they may not like a certain food because it made them sick at one point or they ate it while they were very sick.

Values:
Food selections that may reflect ones religious beliefs, political views or environmental concerns regarding the food the eat or have access to.

FOODS & NUTRIENTS = ENERGY

• Foods are all products we derive from plants and animals that are consumed by the body to provide nutrients and energy for maintenance of life and for the growth and repair of tissues.

• Nutrients are made up of the chemical compounds obtained from our foods and are used by the body to provide us with energy, structural materials and regulating agents to support growth, maintenance and repair of the body's tissues and organs.

• ENERGY is the capacity of the body to do work.
The energy from food is the chemical energy.
The body can convert this chemical energy into mechanical, electrical and heat energy for your use.

The Six Essential Nutrients

The body can manufacture some of its own nutrients, but it cannot make all of the nutrients that are needed or make them in sufficient enough amounts; these nutrients are called essential nutrients.
Essential nutrients must be consumed through your diet in order to meet your body needs.

The body must obtain these nutrients from foods.

Here are the six classes of the essential nutrients:

- Carbohydrates
- Fats/Lipids
- Proteins
- Water
- Minerals
- Vitamins

Macro-nutrients: Carbohydrates, Protein, and Fats

In this section I will tell you why we use the nutrients, exactly what they are used for and educate you on the differences within the nutrient categories.

Carbohydrates

· Types = Simple, Complex and Fiber.
· Primary Function = Supply energy to body.
· Immediate energy source.
· Only fuel usable by both the brain & blood cells.
· Primary fuel for muscles during periods of high intensity exercise.
· Long chains of sugar units.

Simple Carbohydrates

· These are only one to two sugar units in length.
· Monosaccharides & Disaccharides.
· Make the foods you eat sweet.
· Digested and then absorbed quickly which then leads to high-blood glucose levels (larger insulin spikes) and conversion of the food into fat inside the liver.

· Examples= Table sugar, candies, soda/coke, high fructose corn syrup, fruits, honey.

Complex (starchy) Carbohydrates

· Chains of many sugar units (10's to 1000's in length).

· These are Digested and absorbed slowly which then leads to healthy blood glucose levels (or a normal insulin response) and conversion of your food energy for your body.

· Examples=Whole grain, bran, potatoes, oatmeal, wheat/whole grain bread/pastas.

Dietary Fiber

· This is a type of carb, but cannot be digested by the human digestive system, nor does it provide any energy.

· Among its qualities, it helps soften your stool and encourages normal eliminations and healthy bowel movements.

· Fiber rich diets will promote an overall feeling of "fullness", which is quite beneficial for those wanting to drop a few excess pounds.

· Fiber has also been linked to a large reduction in heart attacks, strokes, colon cancer and diabetes.

Two Types of Dietary Fiber:

Soluble

- This type dissolves in water and can be broken down by bacteria in the large intestine.

- Slows down your glucose absorption and then binds up with the cholesterol molecules.

- Sources of soluble fiber include: Fruits, Vegetables, Oats, Barley, Legumes.

Benefits:

- Slower glucose release into your bloodstream.

- Slower stomach emptying and an increased feeling of fullness.

- Reduces absorption of dietary cholesterol by the body.

Insoluble

- This type does not dissolve in water and is not broken down by the bacteria in your large intestine.

- Binds water into your feces....making it softer & bulkier so that it passes quickly & easily through the digestion system.

- Sources of insoluble fiber are: green beans, wheat bran, whole grain breads, whole grain cereals, brussel sprouts.

Benefits:

- Prevents constipation

- Binds up with carcinogens in the body and thereby reducing exposure to them.

BOTH of the forms of fiber will reduce fatty acid absorption and reduce the risk of Colon/Rectal cancer.

However, diets extremely high fiber intake (more than 50 grams per day) can lead to health problems including chronic diarrhea & difficulties with dietary nutrient absorption.

Tips and Recommendations on Carbohydrate Selection

Select foods that are high in fiber like whole grains, oats and bran.

Eat most of your starchy carbs (breads, pastas, cereals, rice, etc) earlier in the day before three PM.

Eat all of your fibrous vegetable carbs
(broccoli, asparagus, spinach, green beans, lettuce, tomato, cucumber, etc)
in place of starchy carbs after three PM.

Limit or cut the intake of simple sugars or sweets, fruit drinks and/or Sodas.

Consume one or two fruit servings every day.

When eating any carbohydrate (simple or complex), it is beneficial to add one to two servings of good fats (almonds, peanut butter, avocado, reduced fat dressing) to reduce insulin release and any spiking.
The fats will bind with carbohydrates in the stomach and release smaller amounts into the intestine. This smaller amount of digested good carbs will indicate a smaller need for the insulin.

Therefore, again reducing chances of excess fat storage.

Proteins

· These nutrients serve as our structural building blocks and they are considered the "work horses" in your body chemistry.

· These are only used for a source of energy when alternative sources are not adequately available, because they're very inefficient to convert to glucose.

Functions of Protein in the Body:

- *Structural Components of Body (Muscle, Bone).*
- *Enzymes (These are the "workhorses" of your body chemistry).*
- *Hormones (communication).*
- *Antibodies (immunity).*
- *Emergency source of energy for the body.*
- *Help maintain your body fluid balance.*

Proteins are made up of nitrogen containing sub-units called "Amino Acids".

There are 20 total amino acids

9 of the 20 amino acids are essential, these are:

Histidine,
Isoleucine,
Phenylalanine,
Methionine,
Leucine,
Threonine,
Valine,
Lysine, and
Tryptophan

Protein Quality: Complete vs. Incomplete

· COMPLETE PROTEINS

- Contain all of the "essential amino acids" and in adequate amounts.
- Good sources include:

Leaner meats, boneless/skinless chicken breasts, fish, egg whites, cheeses, milk, soy......Whey Powder.

· INCOMPLETE PROTEINS

- Lacking one or more of the essential amino acids which creates a Limiting Factor in protein synthesis.

Sources Included: *Oats, Grains, Vegetables, Nuts*

- COMPLIMENTARY PROTEINS

(need to mix & match to get correct quantities and balance).

· Examples:
- *wheat bread/peanut butter*
- *beans/rice*
- *Oats*

Protein Recommendations and selection advice

1. Select lean meats such as tilapia, halibut, boneless/skinless chicken breast or white meat, lean turkey breast, egg whites and whey protein.
Complete proteins are necessary for building lean muscle tissue.
Protein provides 4 calories per gram or 32 calories per gram.

2. Protein needs vary based on activity levels from 0.8 grams per pound body weight in a normal person and 1.2 – 2.2 grams per pound body weight in training athletes.

3. If you are on a high protein diet, it is essential to stay very hydrated. Dehydration and increased protein intake can cause the kidneys to over work themselves.

Fats / Lipids

· These nutrients are our most concentrated source of energy.

· They are a necessary nutrient in the body, however excess should be avoided.

Functions of Fat in Body

- *Storing of Energy.*
- *Absorption of your Fat-Soluble Vitamins.*
- *Adding Flavor & Texture to your Food.*
- *Structural Components of the Hormones.*
- *Structural Components of the Cell Membranes.*
- *Insulation of heat for the Body.*
- *Cushioning of Body.*

Triglycerides

- *95% of all stored lipids in the body*
- *90% of fat weight in foods.*
- *Function = Stored Energy*

Three TYPES of TRIGLYCERIDES

Saturated

- *All of the hydrogen bonding locations are filled.*

- *None of the carbons are double bonded.*

- *More stable so they are solid at room temperature.*

- *usually in red meat, whole milk, cheeses, butter, ice cream.*

- *Causes increases in LDL production or the "bad" cholesterol.*

Monounsaturated

- *All of the hydrogen bonding locations are filled except one.*
- *One pair of the carbons is double bonded.*
- *Sources: olive and canola oil, peanut butter, avocados, almonds.*
- *Reduces total cholesterol, total LDL, and blood triglyceride levels.*
(Reducing risk of heart diseases, strokes, and some cancer)

- *Increases HDL levels -*
MOST EFFECTIVE FOR PROMOTING CARDIOVASCULAR HEALTH

Polyunsaturated

- *There are Multiple hydrogen bonding locations are open.*
- *There are Multiple double bonds are present.*
- *It is Unstable so it is liquid at room temperature.*
- *Sources are Corn & sunflower oils, walnuts, fish, and dark green leafy vegetables.*
- *Reduces total blood cholesterol, blood triglyceride and LDL levels.*
(Reducing your risk of heart diseases, strokes, and some cancer)

There are Two Essential Fatty Acids (and BOTH are polyunsaturated)

Omega-6 Fatty Acids (Also known as: Linoleic Acid)
- *Usual sources include vegetable oils, seeds, nuts, and whole grains.*
- *Usually found in margarine, mayonnaise, and salad dressings.*

Omega-3 Fatty Acids (Also known as: Linolenic Acid)
- *Usual sources are fish and fish oils.*
- *This one is where deficits usually occur in the average diet.*

Functions

- Same as other polyunsaturates, but also has an affect on growth in infants and proper functioning of your nerves and your cell membranes.

Deficits

- Can lead to growth retardation ,as well as, decreased reproductive function & kidney/liver failure.

Fat Selection Tips and Recommendations

You should Select the leanest of fats which are rich in omega-3 and omega-6 fatty acids such as fish oil, olive , canola oil, avocados, almonds, peanut butter, nuts, etc.

Your total calories per day from fats should never be more than 30%.

Not more than 50% of total fats should come from "saturated" sources, such as: *red meats, whole milk, cheese, butter, ice cream.*

Select food low in total overall Cholesterol amounts. 300mg of cholesterol or less per day is okay.

Select Salad dressings which are "Light" and are made with canola oil, olive oil, or safflower oil.

Easy Ways for you to Reduce Fat Consumption

- Prepare meatless main dishes containing smaller amounts of actual meat.
- Remove all skin from chicken & turkey.
- Bake, broil, steam, barbecue, roast, or stew meats. Skip all forms of frying.
- Use lean pieces of meat and make sure to trim off all visible fat.
- Drink non-fat milk.
- Limit use creamier spreads and dressings (substitute vinegarrettes).
- Avoid cooking with lard or oils (use palm & coconut).
- Skim fat off of the top of soups (they naturally dissociate & float at the top).
- Use tomatoes, peppers, onions, garlic, etc. to add flavor to sauces instead of using your butter, creams, or cheeses.

Coconut Oil in our diet plan

Coconut Oil will speed up your metabolism and it produces a decrease in white fat stores, cholesterol and heart disease.
Studies that have added coconut oil to enrich a high fat diet have reported that the coconut oil was effective in producing a reduction of white fat stores.
(Portillo et al, .1998)

Coconut oil really is some amazing stuff.
I definitely prescribe it as definitely one of the most effective and safe ,
as well as, easy to use methods to promote fat loss.
This includes dozens of other fitness-methods and other prescription fat loss drugs.

a.) Coconut Oil will Not Turn To Fat On Your Waist.
Coconut oil is known as a medium chain triglyceride which means it has the shorter molecular chain than your normal fats. Because of this its tendency is to be directly processed in the liver making the chances of coconut oil turning into fat very unlikely.

b.) Coconut Oil Is a Great Source Of Energy.

At 8.3 calories per gram coconut oil has twice the amount of calories as carbohydrates or protein.

Also because coconut oil is a medium chain triglyceride and is absorbed by your liver as fast as straight glucose does. This converts to giving "instant energy". Use of coconut oil in your diet allows you to get more than enough energy in your diet for rigorous training without having to resort
to the use of starchy carbohydrates which love to store as fat.

c.) Coconut Oil and Fractionated Coconut Oil

There are more health benefits to be realized by using natural coconut oil instead of the processed coconut oil.

This is why Fractionated coconut oil is a good choice, but natural unrefined coconut oil is superior and less expensive.

When making shakes or salad dressings, your fractionated oils are the only option .....as they do not solidify at room temperature.

d.) Daily Dosage Recommendation

I recommend eating as much coconut oil as possible during a given day. Using coconut oil as a substitute for butter in as many recipes as you can. This is a good way to lower your chances of gaining weight from the occasional batch of cookies or baked goodies, too.

I also recommend frying using coconut oil.

Many items like eggs will turn out great when coconut oil is used instead.

Carbohydrates choices

Do excess Carbohydrates make You Fat
Or is it the Type of Carbohydrate eaten that make you Fat?

"Low Carb or NO Carbs, Good Carbs or Bad Carbs"
That seems to be the slogan for most "dieters" these days.
Everybody wants a quick fix.
So what do you do?
Who do yo listen to?

Well research has indicated that there are so called "Good Carbs" and "Bad Carbs".
What will help you to distinguish between a good carb or bad carb is what's called the "Glycemic Effect" of food.

What is the "Glycemic Effect" of Food?

The "Glycemic Effect" of food is the measure of the extent to which a food, as it is compared to pure glucose (on a basis of 1 to 100)....will raise blood sugar concentrations and elicit an insulin response.

The "Glycemic Effect" shows us just how quickly glucose can be absorbed for use after a person eats a particular food, how high blood glucose rises, and how quickly it will return back to its normal level.

The best carbs to take in to reduce any form of excessive fat storage are the slow digesting and slow absorbing carbs. The Slow absorbing carbs will give you a low to mild rise in blood glucose with a smooth return to a normal blood glucose level.

In other words.....A low insulin response = low "Glycemic Effect".

Our undesirable carbs produce a "Surge" in blood glucose levels.
This results in a major insulin response followed by an overreaction that plunges blood glucose down. This is what would cause the lethargy or sluggishness you feel after eating a meal with high GI carbs. IE: Thanksgiving Day.

In our day-to-day real life, a food's "Glycemic Effect" differs greatly depending on whether it is eaten alone or as part of a larger meal.
Also, eating frequently, with small meals spreads the glucose absorption throughout the day and thus offers the similar metabolic advantages of eating foods with a low "Glycemic Effect".

This is the reason that using the glycemic index in meal planning is popular with some dietitians, because this type of diet can reduce insulin secretion and improve glucose and fat metabolism.

Additionally, meal plans designed with Low GI foods have also been related to the prevention of heart disease, diabetes and preventing obesity. Slow digesting, high fiber carbs prolong the presence of foods in your digestive track and increase your sensations of fullness and reduce the insulin
response.

The lower your insulin response, equals the less the insulin is produced, which leads to better weight control. In contrast, high GI foods will cause a large insulin response or spike, causing increased cravings, low blood sugar and overeating.

The "Glycemic Effect" of Food is Important for you to Understand

The theory behind the "Glycemic Effect" of Food is to utilize foods From the *Low Glycemic* list of Foods, so that you can support a healthy blood glucose by balancing insulin response naturally.

Your body performs at its best when your blood sugar is kept relatively level and constant. If your blood sugar drops too low, you become lethargic and/or experience an increased hunger, nausea, agitation, headaches and cravings.
On the other hand, if it raises too high, the brain tells your pancreas to secrete more insulin.

Insulin brings your blood sugar back down, however this is done primarily by converting the excess sugar to **stored fat**.

In addition to the high blood glucose is the other fact that the greater the increase in insulin output will drive down blood glucose levels, leading to low overall blood glucose levels....... then the viscous cycle continues unless it is stopped.

Therefore, when eating foods that cause a large and rapid glycemic response, you may feel an initial spike in energy and mood ,as your blood sugar rises, but this will be followed by a cycle of increased storage of fat, lethargy, and extreme food cravings.

How will understanding and then selecting Low GI foods help me Lose Fat?

As has been stated, one of the most effective ways to reduce body fat and control your insulin balance is by eating 5-8 small meals throughout a day. This combined with "physical activity" ,such as resistance training and/or some form of cardio.

Small, frequent meals will also increase the thermic effect of your foods ,as well as, prevent your body from going into its "starvation mode".

Think of it this way..... every time you eat nutrient dense and lower GI foods, your body must burn calories to digest the eaten foods.
Therefore, the more frequently you eat meals, the more you balance your insulin levels and the more calories you burned daily overall.

Many people believe that all they have to do is simply "starve" themselves and they will lose weight.
This is true to some extent. What happens when you do not feed your body?
It will sense a need to preserve itself.

What this does is it slows down its metabolic rate and the body begins to feed on muscle tissue and body fat at a very slow rate.

Even worse, when you decide you want to begin eating again, your metabolic rate is so slow that any excess calorie intake will be stored as,
you guessed it...... body fat.

Current science and research also agrees:

There should be a larger portion of carbohydrates mixed with more moderate amounts of protein and especially fat.
The "Glycemic Index" allows us to more effectively evaluate our nutrition plan, while focusing on the quality of our carbohydrates.

For those of us who incorporate a larger amount of the lower glycemic foods into the diet, we will be rewarded with a more slow and steady release of
glucose; thus keeping insulin levels in check and lowering overall body fat.

Ways to Lower the GI of High GI foods

1. FATS:
Fats slow your gastric emptying and slows the absorption of food.
If absorption into the small intestine is slowed down, the insulin response will be lowered.
Any time you add fats to a meal it will lower the GI of the given meal.

2. FIBER:
Vegetables! Fiber is a complex structure that takes the body a long time to break down and absorb. There are some fiber that is totally indigestible by the body.

The Soluble fibers found in grains, oats, and fruits are ideal.
As they dissolve they tend to gel up in the stomach and Slow down your gastric emptying thereby reducing the insulin response.

3. COMBINING OF CARBS:
You can also lower the total GI of your meal by combining both high glycemic carbs and low glycemic carbs.

For example.... if you ate a baked potato (a High GI) and then ate around the same amount of steamed broccoli (a Low GI), the total GI of the meal would be considerably lower than if you just ate the baked potato alone.

A few facts about the benefits of 'LOW G.I.' foods:

· **B**alancing out your blood sugar levels and reduce the drastic insulin spikes; eat smaller more frequent and balanced meals.

· Each carbohydrate in you eat in meals must be combined with a high quality fat source and some sort of a vegetable.

· You should not have a diet that is too low in fat.
High fat / high protein diets are designed to decrease spikes in insulin and to lower the GI index of foods and your overall meals. Just make sure you are selecting HEALTHY fats such as avocado, peanut butter, almonds, walnuts, low-fat dressings, canola oil and olive oil.

· Low GI diets help people get rid of body fat and control their weight.

· Low GI diets increase your body's sensitivity to insulin.

· Low GI carbs reduce the risk of getting heart disease.

· Low GI carbs reduce the overall blood cholesterol levels.

· Low GI carbs reduce feelings of hunger and keep you fuller for longer periods of time.

· Low GI carbs provide long lasting energy, so you are alert all day long.

Glycemic Index of some Common Foods

For example....If glucose gets a score of 100, what does this actually mean for other foods and their score?

Brown rice is assigned an index number of 55, which then means brown rice raises blood glucose levels 55 percent as much as pure glucose.

In general, any foods below 55 are considered low glycemic index foods, 55-70 represents a midglycemic index food and over 70 are considered higher glycemic foods.

Foods that are Low GI, Moderate GI and High GI:

Low GI (55 or less)

Breads:
100% stone ground whole wheat
Heavy mixed grain
Pumpernickel

Cereal:
All Bran, Bran Buds with Psyllium
Oatmeal, Oat Bran
Muesli

Grains:
Parboiled or converted rice, Barley
Bulgar, Pasta/noodles

Fruits:
Apple, Peaches
Banana, Strawberries
Orange, Grapes

Vegetables:
Broccoli, Lettuce
Cabbage, Mushrooms
Carrots, Green peas

Pastas:
Whole wheat pasta, White spaghetti
Linguini, Macaroni

Rice and Grains:
Brown Rice, White rice
Barely, Buckwheat

Others:
Sweet potato / Yam
Legumes, Lentils
Chickpeas, Kidney beans
Split peas, Soy beans
Baked beans, Fructose
Milk – Whole and Non Fat Yogurt
Honey, Peanuts
Walnuts, Cashews

Medium GI (56-69)

Breads:
Whole wheat Rye
Pita ,Taco shell

Cereal:
Grapenuts, Shredded Wheat
Raisin Bran, Cream of Wheat
Special K

Rice & Grains:
Basmati rice, Couscous
Corn meal

Other:
Potato, new/white Sweet corn
Popcorn, Black bean soup,
Green pea soup

Grains:
Parboiled or converted rice Barley
Bulgar, Pasta/noodles

Fruits:
Papaya, Kiwi
Raisins, Mango
Pineapple

Vegetables:
Corn ,Beets

Pastas:
Whole wheat pasta, White spaghetti, Linguine ,Macaroni

High GI (70 or more)

Breads:
White bread, Kaiser roll
Bagel

Cereal:
Bran flakes, Corn flakes
Rice Krispies and Cheerios

Rice & Grains:
Short-grain rice, Wild Rice
Instant Rice, Glutinous Rice

Other:
Glucose ,Sucrose
Candy ,Gatorade
Soda – Coke, Pepsi
Potato, baking (Russet)
French fries, Pretzels
Rice cakes, Soda crackers
Pancake syrup, Jelly beans

Food Cravings, Lack of Energy and Frequent illness:

Can it be related to stress?
Can this be the reason I gain weight?

Stress has become a popular everyday word in todays society.
How many times has this been said or heard:

" Boy, what a stressful day I just had......"
or
" I have been so stressed-out lately......"

How often do you shovel a sandwich or burger down your throat while typing an e-mail or finishing a report.
Then 15 minutes later feeling bloated, fat and tired?

The term stress describes virtually any alteration or interruption in your life.
It can be physically, emotionally or psychologically.

Most of us recognize stress as a negative feeling ,such as meeting or perhaps a tight deadline for work, financial worries, relationships, or children.
The list goes on and on.

Anxiety of the unknown, fear,anger, frustration and tension are the feelings we also often associate with Stress.

The fact of the matter is, stress can also be experienced from a positive stimulus such as getting married, buying a car or house or witnessing your child graduate from school.
Even when your body responds to an illness, it undergoes some form of inevitable stress.

What you may not realize is that repetitive tension and stress increases the "neuro-chemical response" that clinically has shown to lead to overeating and weight gain.

When your body responds to a stressful situation, it goes through many neuro-chemical, behavior and immunity changes.
These changes are completely out of your control with the goal being to bring your body back to a state of calmness.

It all starts within our brain. When we feel a stress, the brain stimulates our pituitary gland to release a hormone called **"AdrenoCorticotropic Hormone"**
(Also known as **ACTH)**, which then signals the adrenal glands to release various hormones, but mainly adrenaline and cortisol.
Adrenaline makes you feel alert by increasing heart rate and blood pressure.

Adrenaline will also increase your metabolism by the breaking down of fats, carbohydrates and proteins for energy to get the body back to a balanced and happy state. While it is doing this, your body depletes itself of energy stores and the essential vitamins and minerals.

The other hormone which is released is called: **CORTISOL**.

Cortisol is a hormone utilized to breakdown stored energy reserves ,as well as, your muscle tissue.
Cortisol also stimulates release of insulin, which leads to a blood sugar dip and fat storage.

It becomes a vicious cycle that feeds upon itself, over and over until the stress is calmed or gone.

Now that you know that cortisol breaks down stored energy to increase the blood glucose level, which then in turn stimulates insulin secretion.

You can now understand why stress will cause cravings for foods, lethargy, irritability and weight gain.

The sequence of events may appear like this:

1.) Stress response – Assume that your Finances are tight and your bills are due. You have a report due the next day and you will have to miss out on your son's first little league football game. This stressful feeling makes you feel emotions like: fear, anxiety, sweaty palms, etc.

2.) Hormone action – Neuro-chemical reactions cause adrenaline and cortisol to be released. This leads to a rise in blood pressure, heart rate and general alertness.

3.) Action in the body – Breaking down of your stored energy (carbohydrates, fats and proteins) increases your blood glucose levels (which in turn causes insulin to rise) utilizing all blood sugar in you for protection ......leaving you in a LOW BLOOD GLUCOSE State.

4.) LOW BLOOD GLUCOSE – One of the first sure signs of low blood glucose is a craving for candy ,sweets and carbohydrates.
When your blood sugar levels fall lower than normal, symptoms such as nervousness, fatigue, nausea, irritability, depression, disturbed vision, and headaches will begin to appear.

5.) Massive intake of sweets/Candies and refined carbohydrates

6.) The typical human response is now to consume excessive amounts of sweets, junk and refined carbohydrates to feel better and get blood glucose back to normal. The problem with this is the EXCESSIVE intake, which now increases blood glucose too high and spikes yet another insulin response.

This time the insulin response is so drastic that the body stores extra body fat ,from the excessive caloric intake, and then puts the body back into an Low Blood Glucose state again.

7.) Weight Gain and Body Fat storage - Over the long term, A repeat pattern of excessive sugar and refined carbohydrate intake will cause the pancreas to be overworked. With each intake, the pancreas floods the body with insulin, which then makes the blood-sugar level drop dramatically again back to the low blood glucose state and the viscous cycle continues yet again.

The increase in excessive insulin is a major culprit to a weight gain and fat storage.

What if you're still hungry after you finish eating a meal?

If you eat all the recommended protein, carbs, and fat servings for any meal and you are still hungry, we recommend that you eat more green vegetables.

In fact, you can eat unlimited green veggies during every meal. Green vegetables contain low amounts of carbs and high amounts of fiber, which then makes them good for filling you up without all of the added calories.

In order to sufficiently recover from each and every workout and also be ready for your next workout, the proper Workout Nutrition should not be overlooked.

Workout Nutrition is a term we use to describe the nutrients you give your body pre, during, and post workout.

Examples of Supplements so far

Energy Aminos
· Branched Chain Amino Acids (L-Leucine, L-Isoleucine and L-Valine)
· L-Glutamine
· Vitamin B6

During exercise and physical exertion,
Branched Chain Amino Acid (or BCAA's) oxidation......
especially leucine, is increased.

The BCAA's are completely different than the other amino acids in that they are primarily metabolized by the skeletal muscle. So it can meet the increased demand for BCAAs during exercise and physical exertion, the body breaks down muscle tissue to supply any additional BCAA.

By supplying the working body a supplemental BCAA during exercise, you can meet the bodies Increase in demand for BCAA oxidation without breaking down any muscle tissue to supply the needed BCAA.
This leads to greater quality gains in lean muscle tissue and fat loss.

Because the BCAA's serve as the "fuel" for skeletal muscle, BCAA supplementation has been successfully used to enhance sports related performance and recovery.

Whey Protein
· 100% Whey Protein

Coconut Oil

The Blueprint For Your Diet Simplified Serving Breakdowns

Protein per meal

- Less than 150 lbs. = 4 oz. Lean Protein / 4 servings
- 150-200 lbs. = 5 oz. Lean Protein / 5 servings
- over 200 lbs. = 6 oz. Lean Protein / 6 servings

Carbs

- Starchy carbs kept in meals **1, 2 & 3**
- 1-2 Cups of Vegetables per meal
- 2 pieces of fruit per day with meals **4, 5 or 6**

Fats per meal

- Less than 150 lbs. = 2 servings
- 150-200 lbs. = 2-3 servings
- Over 200 lbs. = 3-4 servings

Sample Day consisting of 5 Separate Meals

Meal 1

- **2** servings protein
- 2 servings starchy carbs
- 2 servings fat
- Green Veggies

Meal 2

- **2** servings protein
- 1 serving fruit
- 2 servings fat
- Green Veggies

Meal 3

- **2** servings protein
- 2 servings starchy carbs
- 2 servings fat
- Green Veggies

Meal 4

- **3** servings protein
- 1 serving fruit
- 2 servings fat
- Green Veggies

Meal 5

- **3** servings protein
- **2** servings fat
- Green Veggies

Now Picking Foods and Adding Supplements to the Above Setup
Choose foods from our Approved Foods List

Upon Waking-up
· 1 serving Coffee

Meal 1

· 9 TBSP Egg Whites (3 egg - servings protein)
· 2 Whole Eggs (2 servings protein & 2 fat)
· 1/4 Can Spinach (put in eggs as an omelet)
· 2 pieces Whole Wheat Toast (2 servings carbs)

Meal 2

· 1.5 Scoops Whey Protein (1.5 servings protein)
· 2 TBSP Peanut Butter (2 servings fat)
   A Shake

Meal 3

· 5 oz. Chicken (2 servings protein)
· 2/3 Cups Brown Rice (2 servings carbs)
· 1 Cup Broccoli
· 15-20 Almonds (2 servings fat)

Workout Nutrition
· 1 Scoops Whey Protein

Meal 4
· 1.5 Scoops Whey Protein (2 servings protein)
· 2 TBSP Almond Butter (2 servings fat)

Meal 5
· 5 oz. lean beef (3 servings protein & 1 fat)
· 2 oz. Avocado with added Salsa (2 servings fat)
· 2 Cups Lettuce - All mixed together as a salad

High Performance Nutrient Selection Starches
(equal to 1 serving of Carbohydrate)
12-15 grams carbohydrate

Breads

- Bagel - whole-wheat, oat-bran, 9-grain
- Bread - whole-wheat, oat-bran, 9-grain 1 slice
- Ezekiel bread, 1 slice
- Whole Wheat English muffin ½ or 33g
- Whole Wheat Pita bread (6.5 inch in diameter)
- Whole Wheat Tortilla, 6 inches across 1 or 35g

Cereals & Grains

- Barley (pearled) (dry) 1.25 tbsp or 15.6g
- Kashi Medley 1/3 cup or 19.8g
- Cream of Wheat regular or quick 1.5 tbsp
- Granola, low-fat 2.5 tbsp or 16.5g
- Grape-Nuts 2.5 tbsp or 16.5g
- Honey ¾ tbsp or 15.8g
- Millet (dry) 1.5 tbsp or 18.75g
- Oat Bran (dry) 3.5 tbsp or 20.5g
- Oatmeal (Quaker Instant) ¼ cup or 20g
- Pasta, wheat, (cooked)1/3 cup or 46g
- Quinoa Grain (dry) 1.75 tbsp or 18.6g
- Rice, brown long-grain (cooked) 1/3 cup
- Rolled Oats ¼ cup or 20.25g
- Steel Oats, dry 1/8 cup or 20g

Starchy Vegetables

- Baked potato (no skin) 64g or 2.50 oz
- Baked Sweet potato (baked no skin) 57g
- Yams (baked, no skin) 57g or 2 oz

Dried Beans & Lentils
ALSO COUNTS AS 1 MEAT SERVING

- Black Beans (S&W) 106g or 3.75 oz
- Red Kidney, Pinto Beans (Green Giant)

Fruits
(equal to 1 serving of Carbohydrate)
12-15 grams carbohydrate

- Apple, (with peel) 3.25 oz or 92g
- Banana, (peeled) 2.25 oz or 64g
- Blueberries (fresh) 3.5 oz or 99g
- Grapefruit, (peeled) 6.5 oz or 184g
- Grapes 3 oz or 85g
- Mango (fresh) 3 oz or 85g
- Orange, (peeled) 3.5 oz or 99g
- Pineapple 4 oz or 113g
- Peach (fresh) 4.55 oz or 127.5g
- Pear (fresh) 3 oz or 85g
- Papaya (fresh) 5 oz or 141.75g
- Raisins (seedless) 2 tbsp or 18.5g
- Strawberries (fresh) 6.5 oz or 184g
- Watermelon (fresh) 5 oz or 141.75g

Milk
(equal to 1 serving of Protein & 1 serving Carb)
12-15 grams carbohydrates
6-8 grams protein

Milk & Very Low-Fat Milk
· Skim milk (0 grams fat) 1 cup or 8 Fl oz

· 1% Milk 1 cup or 8 Fl oz

· Plain non-fat yogurt ¾ cup or 6 oz

· Yoplait / Dannon Light Fruit yogurt (1)

Low-Fat Milk
Also Counts as 1 Fat serving
· 2 % milk 1 cup or 8 oz

· Plain low-fat yogurt ¾ cup or 6.5 oz

· Sweet acidophilus milk 1 cup

Whole Milk
Also Counts as 2 Fat servings
· Whole milk 1 cup or 8 oz

Vegetables
(equal to 1 serving of Vegetables)
4-6 grams carbohydrates

· All based on raw or steamed

· Asparagus 4 oz or 113 g

· Broccoli 2.75oz or 78g or ½ cup

· Cauliflower 2.75oz or 78g or ½ cup

· Green Beans 2.2oz or 62.5g or ½ cup

· Onions 53g or 1.86 oz or 1/3 cup

· Spinach 125g or 4.4oz or 2/3 cup

· Celery 120g or 4.25 oz or 1 cup

· Cucumber 156g or 5.5 oz or 1/3 cup

· Green onions 50g or 1.75 oz or ½ cup

· Mushrooms 78g or 2.5 oz or ½ cup

· Tomato 90g or 3.2 oz or ½ cup

· Salad greens (lettuce, romaine) 3 cups

Protein
(equal to 1 serving of Meat)
6-8 grams protein

Very Lean Meats
(all measurements AFTER cooked)

· Chicken breast boneless/skinless 1 oz

· Turkey breast (LEAN) 1 oz or 28.35g

· Fresh fish (cod, halibut, tuna, tilapia) 1 oz

· Shell fish (crab, lobster, shrimp or ?) 1.25 oz

· Egg whites 2 or 67g

· Egg Beaters ¼ cup or 2.15 oz or 61g

· Non-fat cottage cheese at ¼ cup

· Salmon Fillet 1 oz or 28.35g (also ½ fat)

· Lean Sirloin ¾ oz or 21.25g

· Egg (including yolk) 1 or 50g (also 1 fat)

· Cheese 2% (Reduced Fat) 1 oz or 28.35g (1 fat)

· Salmon 1 oz or 28.35g (also counts as ½ fat serving)

Fat (equal to 1 serving of Fat)
5 grams fat

Monounsaturated Fats & Polyunsaturated Fats

· Avocado 1 oz or 28.35g

· Almonds (dry roasted) 1/3 oz (~ 6 pieces) or 1 tbsp

· Cashews 1/3 oz or 1 tbsp or 9.65g

· Mayonnaise (Light, reduced-fat) 1 Tbsp or 15g

· Oil (olive or canola) 1 tsp or 4.5g or 0.16 oz

· Peanuts 1/3 oz or 9.36g

· Peanut/Almond butter (smooth or crunchy) 2 tbsp

· Pecans ¼ oz or 1 tbsp or 7.44g

· Salad dressing (Light, reduced-fat) 2 Tbsp or 30g

· The right Light spread 1 tbsp or 14g

· Sunflower seeds 1Tbsp or 1/3 oz or 9.0g

· Walnuts 1Tbsp or 1/4 oz or 7.5g

Free Food List

Less than 20 calories per serving
Less than a 5 gram serving of carbohydrate
Recommended to be at : 1 serving per meal per day

Fat Free or Reduced Fat

- Cream cheese 1 Tbsp
- Creamers, non-dairy liquid 1 Tbsp
- Creamer, non-dairy powder 2 Tbsp
- Mayonnaise, fat-free 1 Tbsp
- Margarine, fat-free 4 Tbsp
- Miracle Whip, non-fat 1 Tbsp
- Salad dressing, fat-free 1 Tbsp
- Sour cream, fat-free 2 Tbsp

Sugar Free or Low Sugar

- Hard candy, sugar free 1 piece
- Gelatin dessert, sugar free 1
- Gum, sugar free 1 piece
- Jam or jelly. Low sugar or light 2 tsp
- Syrup, sugar free 2 Tbsp

Drinks

- Coffee
- Club soda
- Diet soft drinks, sugar free
- Tea

Sugar Substitutes

- Equal (aspartame)
- Splenda (Sucralose)
- Sprinkle Sweet (saccharin)
- Sweet One (Acesulfame potassium)
- Sweet 'n Low (saccharin)

When do I eat for training?

We recommend eating first thing in the morning to get the body cranking right away.
Breakfast is the most important meal all day.
So....Get up, wash your face, go to the bathroom and then start making breakfast.

As for scheduling your training, we recommend planning your meals so that one of your meals (preferably a Meal Shake) falls 90 minutes before you workout (the PRE-WORKOUT MEAL) and then the next meal would be scheduled to fall 60 minutes after the workout.

I also recommend a "whey protein shake" immediately following any workout.

Then within 60 minutes, eat your next scheduled meal.
Every meal thereafter should be two to four hours apart.

If you get up at 6am and train in the morning then your meals would look like this:

6:00 AM - Meal 1

7-8:30 AM - Workout

9:00 AM - Meal 2

12:00 PM - Meal 3

4:00 PM - Meal 4

8:00 PM - Meal 5

If you get up at 6am and train in the evening then your meals will look like this:

6:00 AM - Meal 1

9:00 AM - Meal 2

12:00 PM - Meal 3

3:00 PM - Meal 4

6-7:30 PM - Workout

8:30 PM - Meal 5

Setting Up Your Own Diet

Your goal is to get 5-8 small sized meals per day.
Depending upon caloric intake per day.
Eating small, frequently spaced meals will help to keep blood glucose and insulin levels stable and keeps you full and satisfied while promoting the desired fat loss.

Your Protein Intake

Your diet is geared towards making the "dieting" less complicated so you can live your life less restricted. Instead of getting bogged down with counting each and every single gram of protein or calorie from your diet and trying to hit an exact amount each day, we simplify things & recommend eating 4-6 oz. of a lean protein source each meal.

1 oz. of lean meat equals about 7 grams of protein, so you will be obviously eating 28-42 grams of protein per meal.

Good proteins include the usuals: chicken, lean beef and turkey, tuna and the other fish, Whey protein and also egg whites.

Your Carbohydrate Intake

Your diet is designed as a low carbohydrate diet, structured to maintain stable insulin and blood sugar levels.

Our carbohydrate intake recommendation is actually simple. 1-2 cups of green vegetables with each meal and 2-3 pieces of fruit per day eaten with meals.

Each cup of vegetables contains roughly 10grams of carbohydrates.

A meal that contains 1 cup of vegetables and 1 piece of fruit will have about 30 grams of carbohydrates in it.

Your Fat Intake

Dietary fat is very important for proper body maintenance and functioning. Most people have an unbalanced knowledge of dietary fat and therefore limit or cut it completely.

Your diet promotes getting your good fats with each and every meal, which helps to maintain stable blood glucose and insulin levels.

We recommend that you get 10-20 grams of fat with each meal.

Good sources of fat include:

almonds and almond butter
peanuts and peanut butter
avocado
flax seed
olive oil and
of course..... coconut oil.

Your Carb Refeed / Cheat Meal

We recommend a carb refeed meal every three days or so.

In the diet we give you the option of having yourself a "cheat" meal in place of the carb refeeds, which will allow you to go out to eat with your friends and family and/or just enjoy yourself while not hampering any of your progress.

While we recommend eating good complex carbs like grains
(such as oatmeal) and starches (such as sweet potatoes) for your carb refeed, certainly a couple slices of pizza or candy at the movies every now and then will not kill your progress and allows you to enjoy life.

<u>"Cheating"</u>

How much can I cheat?

Let's set forth a few guidelines here. While it is okay having the occasional Thanksgiving day-like feast where you eat until your pants don't fit and your feet are swollen, we obviously do not recommend doing this on a weekly basis.

Thus, when you are following the aforementioned diet program, we recommend two to three cheat meals every week with calories at somewhere around 150% of your normal meal. Meaning that if a normal meal for you averages 500 calories, you will allow the cheat meal to be somewhere around 750 calories or so.
But how do you expect to count the cheating calories?

You won't. It is all about moderation and approximating the your actual total. In essence, eat until you are full, but definitely not until you are stuffed.

What can I eat for my cheat meal?

We obviously recommend making healthiest of choices, but the beauty of the cheat meal is that you can cave-in to those cravings!
If you feel like a piece of pie then get a big slice of Pecan Pie.
If you feel like cheese then buy a big cheddar loaf!
Just control yourself and not eat the whole pie or an entire loaf of cheese.
The beauty is that you can kiss those protein,carb and fat ratios goodbye for this meal.
Enjoy!

What about after I have cheated? Should I not eat the rest of the day?

You will need to Eat your next scheduled meal after the cheat session.
If you Are way too full to do this, simply skip the meal (try not to do this) or eat a portion of your next scheduled meal.
Maybe a piece of fruit?

What about after that?

If you feel you went overboard on the cheating, you can then add five or ten minutes of extra cardio to the next two to three cardio sessions.

If the day after the cheat meal is an off day from your training, you can do an extra 20 to 30 minutes of easy cardio cardio. Outlined in your Cardio Program.

Bringing it all together

The goal is to add and subtract items in and out of your diet over the course of time.

This way we can eliminate foods that dont react well with your body and /or lifestyle.

Most people dont even know they have a "Food Allergy" or bad reaction to foods; until they really experiment a little bit and realize that even the thought of eating a particular food adds 5 pounds!

We are also starting to experiment with new supplements and diet timing.....This way we can learn how to keep your body always in an anabolic/fat burning state; while not feeding it foods that it hates and that seem to pack on fat.

4. Your Strategic Shake Diet

Meal Replacement Shakes

Shakes are a very innovative way of building your own rapid weight loss or muscle building program.

Also known as meal replacement shakes, they are designed to easily replace your daily meals.

There are several different shake recipes intended for weight loss or gain, but the most common variant is the generic "protein diet shake".

Hundreds of clients and athletes have testified to the value of this particular tool for anyone desiring to lose or gain weight using natural methods.

Drinking prepared "meal shakes" as your diet staple offer a lot of amazing health benefits. While making it totally simple and virtually fool proof.
It is also the most cost-friendly way to diet.

A meal replacement shake provides you with the best and the most important nutrients and energy to perform your upcoming daily activities.
Even better, it helps to stabilize your blood sugar levels, which is the key factor if you intend to consume meal replacement shakes as part of your diet.

As soon as your blood sugar level drops, you begin to have cravings for foods that could ruin your weight loss efforts.

You must also take note of the calorie content in your shake to ensure that you are not sabotaging your entire diet and nutritional goal.
The recommended amount of calories for your meal replacement shake should be between 50% and 75% per day.

What you need to remember is that this is **NOT** a "diet supplement", but is a replacement for and still **is a meal**. So it has to contain enough calories and whole foods to meet your body's daily requirements.

To get the real benefit of using diet shakes as meal replacement, you must apply them as an alternative to 3-6 meals each day.

In our program, we suggest breakfast(s) and we suggest lunch(s).
Also the bedtime shake and post-workout shake with a Protein/low carb version.

One reason is that most people are most active during the daytime, so it makes sense that you will easily burn off excess fat during the busiest part of the day.

At night while you sleep, as we learned, is when the body repairs itself.
Hence the Protein only shake before bed.

For a healthier rapid weight loss diet alternative, carefully choose the food sources for preparing your shake.
Some of the best known protein sources would be egg whites, whey protein , or soy protein.

The liquid component of your shakes depend on your own preference.....Rice milk, soy milk, almond milk, fat-free milk or water.

You can add sweeteners like honey or frozen fruit to make it pleasant tasting and to ensure that you enjoy consuming this while you are losing weight at the same time.

Carbohydrates may be replaced by fruits, oats and/or sweet potatoes.
(See more of the diet section for suggested foods and use common sense here)

The ability to enjoy great tasting food or beverages while shedding off excess fat is the ultimate source for your weight loss answers.

Over time....The size of the stomach will begin to decrease or shrink.
This achieves the same results as the surgical procedures, but at no cost, and is reversible.

Nine Protein Shake Recipes

- If instructions are not supplied, assume you should blend all ingredients together for approximately one minute.

1. **The Lite Shake**

Ingredients & Instructions:
- 1 cup fat-free skim milk
- 1 scoop Whey protein
- a little bit of crystal light to match
- 1 teaspoon coconut oil

2. **Banana Meal Milk Shake**

Ingredients & Instructions:
- 1 banana
- 2 cups fat-free milk
- 2cups water
- 1 tsp. "Super Greens" (see appendix)
- 1 scoop Whey protein powder
- 2 tbsp. Honey and coconut oil
- 1 yogurt (optional)
- Mix in blender.

3. Chocolate Peanut butter meal

Ingredients & Instructions:
- 3 cup fat-free milk
- 2 tblsp peanut butter / almond butter
- 2 tblsp Honey and coconut oil
- 1 tblsp "Super Greens"
- 2 scoopfuls of whey chocolate protein

4. Super Carb Meal Shake

Ingredients & Instructions:
- 3 cups water
- 1/2 a peeled grapefruit
- 1 tblsp Honey and coconut oil
- Crystal light accordingly

5. Frozen Chocolate Banana

Ingredients & Instructions:
- 1.5 cups each Water and fat-free milk
- 4 ice cubes
- 1 banana
- 1 tblsp of "Super Greens" and Coconut oil
- 2 scoopfuls of whey chocolate protein

6. German Chocolate Cake

Ingredients & Instructions:
- 1.5 cups each water and fat-free milk
- 4 ice cubes
- 1 tablespoon coconut oil
- 1 cap of "cream of coconut"
- 2 scoopfuls of whey chocolate protein

7. Tangerine Cream

Ingredients & Instructions:
- 12 oz. Tangerine Diet Rite
- 4 Ice Cubes
- 1 tblsp of coconut oil
- 1.5 scoops of vanilla whey protein

8. Root Beer Float

Ingredients & Instructions:
- 1 can Diet A&W Root Beer
- 1 tblsp of coconut oil
- 4 ice cubes
- 1.5 scoops of vanilla whey protein

9. Pineapple Carb Blast

Ingredients & Instructions:
- 1 tblsp coconut oil
- 3 cups water
- Crystal light accordingly
- 1/2 cup pineapple chunks

18 Foods to Mix-in with your Shakes

1. Fat-Free Milk - Just use the milk instead of water for more flavor, richness, thickness, and more protein and calories.

2. Powder milk - Use this for a lot more flavor, carbs, protein and calories.

3. Fruit - Blend all this up and it's called a "fruit smoothie".
We can try strawberries, blueberries and bananas.
Add the fruit to just about all of these recipes. Fruits add Tons of vitamins, a lot of minerals, gobs of fiber and anti-oxidants; so don't hesitate adding them.

4. Nuts/Legumes - Mix and/or blend with walnuts, almonds, and pecans. Will add Some healthy fats to it and a bit of a nutty aftertaste to everything.

5. Peanut or Almond Butter –
Use as an addition of carbs, fats and healthy protein.

6. Oatmeal - You can make strawberry or chocolate protein oatmeal for your high fiber / High protein breakfast. Just add 1/4 cup of raw oatmeal to a plain chocolate or strawberry protein shake.

7. Cereal - Breakfast Cereals are generally not too good for diet or you, unless you're eating something like a Total, Special K, Grapenuts, or Kashi; and that's exactly what I'm recommending here. Add a scoop or two of protein powder and your healthy cereal and the milk and hit BLEND!

8. Cottage Cheese – Use 1/4 cup at the most. Add fruit and nuts as desired.

9. Coconut Oil -
1 gram per shake. See the section regarding this awesome stuff

10. Frozen Yogurt – Blend in one cup. Adds extra protein, Calories and taste.

11. Pudding Mix – You can make a protein low-fat pudding with virtually any flavor of pudding or protein. Mix protein, Whey and milk. Blend. Chill.

12. Apple Juice and Caramel Flavoring – Mix it with a vanilla whey protein for a Caramelled apple dessert shake. Add fruit and nuts as desired.

13. Other Juices – You can also use virtually any other juice.
Try orange juice, cranberry juice, or any other juice you like.

14. Yogurt - Low-fat or non-fat yogurt mixed with fruit or even just a vanilla flavored. Blend it with fruit and whey powder for an awesome fruit smoothie. Add fruit and nuts as desired.

15. Egg Whites – Separate yolks from eggs. ....Maybe 4 to 6 eggs. Microwave for 30 to 45 seconds
(NO RAW EGGS!)

16. Mashed Potatoes or Sweet Potatoes – Blend in for a major dose of carbs, calories, starchy carbs and vitamins

17. Sweeteners - Add any type of syrup if you're not too worried about extra carbs, and add any type of artificial sweetener (I prefer Crystal Lite) if you want to avoid sweetening your protein with sugar and are concerned about extra carbs and calories. Coffee flavorings work well also.

18. Coffee – Mix up a scoop of chocolate protein with milk, then add the milk and then add the two cups of coffee.

Bringing it all together

The shakes are designed to replace meals.
Usually 1 or 2 meals per day.
We are doing this mainly so we can fit Super-Foods into your diet without having to go through all of the eating and time required to do so.

Actually EATING 6 or 7 meals a day is hell!
Drinking 2 cups of "Shake" with everything neatly and conveniently packed/hidden away.....Is simple!
Plus....The forced use of ACTUAL "Servings" in shake perpetration ends up saving a huge amount of money.
My current diet level has 3/4 of my nutrition coming from "Shakes".
It costs me $60 to make a months supply of "mix" PLUS the eggs and sweet potatoes.
So MAYBE $100 a month in food costs on a controlled "Bodybuilder Diet".

The long-term effects of the shake diet are a "Shrunken stomach".....
whereby the stomach actually shrinks and makes it possible to "fill up" on less food....which is then spaced out and eaten evenly during the day.

5. Your 100 Shake Recipes

The Best Protein Shake Ever
1 scoops Chocolate Whey Powder
10 Ice Cubes
2 cups of fat-free milk
2 table spoon fat-free vanilla yogurt or Kefir
1 table spoon reduced fat peanut butter
2 table spoon hazelnut coffee
1/8 cup caramel ice cream topping

Lean Mass Banana Split Shake
1/2 fresh banana
2 tablespoon Whipping cream (heavy cream, not cream out of a can)
2 Scoops Chocolate Whey Powder
2 cups of water
4-6 ice cubes

Heavy Gainer Protein Shake
1 scoop Chocolate Whey Powder
2 egg whites
1 tablespoon Peanut Butter
2 cups cold water
2 cups ice

Banana Bread Shake
Ingredients:
1 scoop Vanilla Whey Powder
1 Banana
1/2 Cup Rolled Oatmeal (cook with boiling water) or Bran
3/4 Cup Kellogg's Bran Flakes
1 cups of water
Sugar, Brown Sugar or Stevia Sweetener to taste

Banana Protein Shake
Ingredients:
1 scoop Vanilla Whey Powder
1 medium to large banana
2 cups low-fat Milk
1 tablespoon Linseed, Soy and Almond Mixture
1 teaspoon Golden Syrup
Few drops vanilla essence/extract
3-4 cubes ice
1 tablespoon low-fat natural yogurt

Orange Vanilla Shake
Ingredients:
1 scoop of Vanilla Whey Powder
2 cups of Orange Juice
4-5 ice cubes
1 teaspoon Vanilla Extract
½ banana
2-3 fresh strawberries
2 packets of sweetener

Protein-Carb Almond Protein Shake Blaster
Ingredients:
1 scoop Vanilla Whey Powder
2 cups of skim milk
1 cup of dry oatmeal
1 cup of raisins
12 shredded almonds
1 tablespoon of peanut butter

Plum Ice Shake
Ingredients:
1 scoop Vanilla Whey Powder
1 ripe plum (pitted) juice of 1 lemon
2 cups of ice water
1.2 cup of ice cubes

Plum-Lemon Cooler
Ingredients:
1 scoop Vanilla Whey Powder
1 ripe plum, pitted
juice of 1 lemon
1 multi-vitamin
2 cups ice water
1/2 cup ice cubes

Wild Berry Boost
Ingredients:
2 scoops Vanilla Whey Powder
8 raspberries
4 strawberries
15 blueberries
3 cups of non-fat milk
1/2 cup ice cubes

Creatine Catalyst
Ingredients:
1 scoop Vanilla Whey Powder
5 Granny Smith apples
5 grams (one teaspoon) Creatine powder
1/2 cup ice cubes and 2 cups water

Peanut Brittle Protein Shake
Ingredients:
2 scoops vanilla protein
1 tablespoon sugar-free instant butterscotch pudding mix, dry
1 tablespoon natural peanut butter, chunky
2 cups of cold water or low-fat milk
3-6 ice cubes

The Hulk Protein Shake
Ingredients:
1 scoop vanilla protein
1 tablespoon sugar-free pistachio pudding mix
1 mint leaf or a few drops peppermint extract
1 tablespoon green tea
1 few drops green food coloring (optional)

1 cups of cold water or low-fat milk
3-5 ice cubes

Oatmeal Meal Replacement Shake

Ingredients:
1 cup dry measure oatmeal, cooked in water and cooled
2 scoops vanilla protein
3 dashes cinnamon
1/8 cup sugar-free maple syrup or equivalent amount brown sugar
1 tablespoon chopped almonds (or flaxseed oil or natural peanut butter)
2 cups of water or low-fat milk

Cinnamon Roll Protein Shake

Ingredients:
1 scoop vanilla Whey Powder
1 tablespoon sugar-free instant vanilla pudding
1/4 teaspoon cinnamon
1/2 teaspoon imitation vanilla (or 1/4 teaspoon extract)
1 packet artificial sweetener
a few dashes butter flavor sprinkles or butter-flavor extract
2 cups water (or low-fat milk)
3 ice cubes

Nada Colada Protein Shake
Ingredients:
1 scoop vanilla Whey Powder
1/2 cup of pineapple and/or orange juice
1/4 teaspoon rum extract
1/4 teaspoon coconut extract (or 2 tablespoon shredded coconut)
1 packet artificial sweetener
4 ounce water (or low-fat milk)
3-6 ice cubes

Tropical Treat
Ingredients:
2 cups of water
1/2 banana (fresh)
2 teaspoon low-fat sour cream
1 teaspoon coconut extract
1 scoop Vanilla Whey Powder

Super Healthy Honey Banana Shake
2 cups of water
1 big scoop of vanilla Whey Powder
3/4 cup of natural yogurt
1 banana
1 teaspoon of flax seed oil
2 teaspoon of honey
1 teaspoon Spirulina

Rock N' Roll Protein Shake
Ingredients:
2 cups of water
1 scoop of vanilla Whey Powder
3/4 cup of natural yogurt
1 banana
1 teaspoon of flax seed oil
2 teaspoon of honey
1 teaspoon Spirulina

Pineapple Protein Shake Power
Ingredients:
1 cup of pineapple juice
3 strawberries
1 banana
1 teaspoon of yogurt
1 scoop of your choice of protein

Strawberry Protein Shake Savior
Ingredients:

4 scoops vanilla Whey Powder
2 cups of water
1 strawberry yogurt
3 fresh strawberries
1 teaspoon creatine
1 teaspoon flax seed oil

Vanilla Coffee Delight
Ingredients:
2 cups low-fat milk
1 scoops vanilla Whey Powder
1/2 cup low-fat coffee flavored ice cream

Vanilla Egg Heavy Gainer
Ingredients:
1 scoop Whey Powder Vanilla
2 egg whites
1 tablespoon Peanut Butter
1 cup water cold water
2 cups ice

Peanut Butter And Banana Shake
Ingredients:
1 scoop Whey Protein
Small handful almond flakes
1 tablespoon peanut butter
2 cups skim milk
half of a banana
1 tablespoon honey

The Best Overall Tasting Homemade Protein Shake
Ingredients:
16 ounce skim milk
2 cups no-fat cottage cheese
3 scoops vanilla Whey Powder
1/2 cup non-fat, reduced-sugar vanilla yogurt scoop of your favorite fruit
(I like fresh strawberries & banana)
Handful of Ice

PB&J Protein Shake
1 Scoops Vanilla Whey Powder
8-12 ounce water (add 1% milk if you want a little creamier texture)
1 tablespoon Natural (smooth) Peanut Butter
1 tablespoon Flax oil or Flax meal
1 teaspoon sugar-free Strawberry Jam

Fruity Carbohydrate High Protein Shake – (Post or Pre-Workout)
1 banana (cut in pieces and fresh)
4-6 whole strawberries
1/2 cup low-fat yogurt
2 cup orange or pineapple juice
1 scoop Vanilla Whey Powder

Tropical Protein Pina Colada Shake
1 scoop Vanilla low carb Whey Powder
2 cups of water
1/3 cup pineapple chunks – freeze them for icy texture
Coconut milk or coconut extract
1/2 cup 2% milk + 1/2 cup pineapple
4-6 ice cubes

Root Beer Float
12 ounce can of diet Root Beer
1 scoops Vanilla Whey Powder
4-6 ice cubes
2 tablespoon Whipping cream (heavy cream, not from a can)

Mango Madness
1 scoop Vanilla Whey Powder
1/2 to 1 cup mango pieces fresh or freshly sliced natural mango
1 cup Vanilla yogurt
1 tablespoon Flax seed oil
3 cups of water

Dreamsicle Protein Shake
1 Scoops Vanilla Whey Powder
Seeds from half a length of real vanilla bean
1 teaspoon Vanilla extract
3 cups of water
1 peeled orange
3 tablespoon Whipping cream (heavy cream, not from can)
1/2 cup vanilla yogurt
Ice cubes at end to add desired consistency

Mineral Power
3 cups of water
1 scoop of "Super Greens" or similar
1 packet gelatin
1 teaspoon flax seed oil
1 big scoop of vanilla Whey Powder

Rock N' Roll Protein Shake
1 cup of water
1 scoop of vanilla Whey Powder
3/4 cup of natural yogurt
1 banana
1 teaspoon of flax seed oil
2 teaspoon of honey
1 teaspoon Spirulina

Strawberry Savior
1 scoops vanilla Whey Powder
8 fluid ounces water
1 strawberry yogurt
3 fresh strawberries
1 teaspoon creatine
1 teaspoon flax seed oil

Vanilla Coffee Delight
2 cups low-fat milk
1 scoops vanilla Whey Powder
1/2 cup low-fat coffee flavored ice cream

Peanut Butter And Banana Shake
1 scoop vanilla Whey Powder
small handful almond flakes
1 tablespoon peanut butter
3 cups skim milk
Half a banana
1 tablespoon honey

The Best Overall Tasting Homemade Protein Shake
16 ounce skim milk
2 cups no-fat cottage cheese
3 scoops vanilla Whey Powder
1/2 cup non-fat, vanilla yogurt scoop of your favorite fruit
Handful of Ice

Ginger Bread Man
1 scoop vanilla Whey Powder
1 graham cracker
1/2 teaspoon cinnamon
vanilla extract
12ounce of water
4 Ice Cubes

Creamy Coffee Ice Cream
1 scoop vanilla Whey Powder
13 ounce ice cubes
3 ounce water
2 teaspoon ground coffee

Apple Pie Delight
1 scoop vanilla Whey Powder
1 peeled and cored apple, cut into pieces
2 cups of milk
1/2 teaspoon cinnamon
1/2 teaspoon nutmeg
5 Ice Cubes

Holiday Pumpkin Spice Shake (low carb/ diet shake)
2 Scoops Vanilla Whey Powder
8 ounce water
1 tablespoon Flax oil
1teaspoon Pumpkin pie spice
8 ounce Yogurt
4-6 ice cubes

Fruit Smoothie
2 scoops Strawberry Whey Powder
4 large strawberries
blueberries (a small handful)
water (just a few drops)
1/2 Cup of ice

Egg Full Shake
3 eggs
3 cup milk
1 scoop Whey Protein

Tropical Pleasure
Ingredients:
8 ounce pure water
1/2 teaspoon pineapple extract
1/2 teaspoon coconut extract
1 tablespoon heavy cream
1/2 fresh banana
1 heaping scoop (1 ounce) of Egg Protein
2-3 ice cubes (optional)

Eggcellent Protein Shake
Ingredients:
3 eggs

1 cup milk or 3-4 scoops vanilla ice cream
Add all ingredients in blender. Blend and enjoy.

Banana Almond Creme
Ingredients:
1 Banana
2 Cup Milk
10 Almonds
1 Serving Protein
5 Ice Cubes

Chocolate Coffee Shake
Ingredients:
Mix 2 scoops of Milk Chocolate Protein
1 cup of skim milk
5 ice cubes
1 cup of water
1 spoonful of instant coffee

Peppermint Oatmeal Shake
Ingredients:
Mix 2 scoops of Milk Chocolate Protein
1 cup sugar-free vanilla ice cream
1 cup oatmeal
2 cups non-fat milk
1 cup water
a splash of peppermint extract

Banana Almond Creme
1 Banana
2 Cup Milk
10 Almonds
1 Serving Protein
5 Ice Cubes

Snickers® Meal Replacement Shake
3 Mini Snickers® Bars
4 eggs
3 cups milk
2 tablespoons evaporated milk
Chop the candy into cubes. Add the milk, eggs, then mix; add the evaporated milk and mix.

Protein Bars Shake
3 Protein Bars
4 eggs
3 cups milk
2 tablespoons evaporated milk
Chop the Protein Bars into cubes. Add the milk, eggs, then mix; add the evaporated milk and mix.

Muscle Shake
1 cup low-fat milk
1/2 cup plain low-fat yogurt
1 banana, sliced
2 tablespoon Whey Powder
6 strawberries, sliced
1 teaspoon wheat germ
1 tablespoon honey or maple syrup

1/4 cup of any fresh berries
Pinch of nutmeg or carob powder

Mineral Power
Ingredients:
10 ounce pure water
1 ounce liquid ionic plant source minerals
1 teaspoon flax-seed oil
1 heaping scoop (1 ounce) of protein of choice

Weight Gainer
14 ounce pure water
2 bananas or 2 scoops YAM Power
3 teaspoon peanut butter
1 scoop of your choice of protein

Pineapple Power
1 cup of pineapple juice
3 strawberries
1 banana
1 teaspoon of yogurt
1 scoop of your choice of protein

Banana Delight
Ingredients:
8 ounce pure water
1/2 banana (fresh)
2 ounce protein of choice
2 teaspoon flax seed

Strawberry Cheesecake
Ingredients:
10 ounce pure water
8 fresh strawberries
4 teaspoon low-fat sour cream
1.5 ounce protein of choice

Blueberry Dream
Ingredients:
10 ounce Pure water
1/2 cup fresh or fresh blueberries
1.5 ounce protein of choice
2 teaspoon flax seed

Peaches and Sour Cream
Ingredients:
8 ounce pure water
1 ripe peach
2 teaspoon low-fat sour cream
1.5 scoop protein of choice

Quick Start
3 cups water
3 oranges
1 ounce protein of choice

High Energy Shake!
Ingredients:
10 ounce pure water
10 strawberries (Fresh or fresh)
1 teaspoon flax seed
1/2 teaspoon Green Tea Powder
1/2 teaspoon vanilla extract
1 heaping scoop of protein of choice
2-3 ice cubes (optional)

Super Slimmer
Ingredients:
8 ounce pure water
1 teaspoon flax seed
1/2 ripe peach (peeled)
6 fresh strawberries
1 heaping scoop of protein of choice

Heavy Gainer
Ingredients:
10-14 ounce pure water
1/2 cup raw almonds – blend with water only until creamy smooth then add…

1/2 large fresh banana
2 level scoops (2 ounce) of protein of choice

Weight Gainer
Ingredients:
3 cups pure water
2 bananas or 2 scoops YAM
3 teaspoon peanut butter
2 ounce protein of choice

6. Your Supplementation

Here are the top 8 supplements

No matter what sport you choose, athletes are always after one thing: winning. To win, you typically have to be a better athlete and we all know.... a better athlete is one who is faster, stronger, better prepared and with superior training. The next question should be..... how does one achieve all of those before mentioned winning goals?

First of all, it requires dedication both on and off of the field. In and outside of the gym. There is no way to prepare for any particular sport without required practice and then there is no way to be successful without intensive practice.

Therefore, one must eat correctly to properly fuel the body, He or she must get sufficient rest for recovery and also put in some extra time in the weight room or etc to get stronger.

If all of those things are in order, THEN we may consider dietary supplements.

This issue should not go without a bit of background research; I have talked with way too many people who are taking dozens of different supplements and can not tell me what any of them are actually for. Or, if they can tell me what they are for, they have no idea why they are taking it or how much they are or should be taking.

If you are going to take any dietary supplement, do some research and understand what it is supposed to do for you and figure out the actual recommended dose. Next, never introduce your body to more than one supplement at a time. I say this because if you dont .....then you won't know if one is working or not.

Here is a great example of a situation I encountered. I was talking with a collegiate football player who had decided he was going to start using glutamine. He told me he had also started taking creatine, protein, a recovery drink, a Pre-workout, BCAA's and also a meal replacement. At the same time, he had also made some large dietary changes and had just went into a strength phase of his weight training workouts.

Two weeks later, he was telling me all about how they had all worked great because he noticed tremendous changes both in and out of the gym.

The question I then asked him was.......

"exactly what caused those changes?"

He quickly responded................

"the creatine works great and so do the other supplements."

The only problem is that there is absolutely no way he could have known if any of the supplements had in fact worked for him. How can he know or not whether it wasn't that he had merely started eating more calories? Or because he was now training quite differently? If it was actually only ONE supplement working and the 3 others were actually subtracting negatively from its lone success?

If you want to start taking creatine, for an example, do not change anything else about your current diet, workout regimen, or supplement your protocol. Solely add creatine to your daily routine and begin to assess the changes.....if any.

This will allow you to decipher where any positive changes are coming from.

With all that now said, here are my top 8 supplements that you might consider...........

1.) Multivitamin / mineral

While this is may sound a little "boring" it needs to be the cornerstone of any supplement regimen. For those who are currently eating a sound and well balanced diet, it will merely act as an "insurance policy". It is not necessary to have any massive doses of any vitamin or mineral....... your basic multi-vitamin from the corner store is fine.

2.) Whey Protein Powder

This is great for convenience. However, you should not live off of the powder. I've talked to some athletes who were consuming up to 6 a day. When making a shake, add some frozen fruit as a way to get more fruit into the diet.

We have this subject covered thoroughly in other chapters.

3.) Meal Replacement Bar

Similar to meal replacement powders, these are also good for convenience. These are great for your locker or the car...... so there is always something available to eat.

I would much rather have you eat one of these (or a shake) than stop at the most convenient fast food restaurant drive-thru window everyday.

4.) Creatine

There is absolutely plenty of documented research to support the claims of this supplement. Remember that more is not better, so do not exceed the recommendations prescribed. It's roughly 5 grams every 24 hours. In fact, recent research demonstrates that it may only take 3 grams/day to saturate muscles (less than the 5 grams typically recommended).

5.) Fish Oil

There is sufficient documented research to support your use of fish oil for cardiovascular health. There is also quite a bit of research to support the use of fish oil for reducing inflammation. This is important when you are recovering from your grueling workouts and healing from your ailments. Try 1-2 grams per day.

6.) Flax Oil

Similar to the fish oil, this is also a healthy fat that should become an important component of the athletes diet. The majority of American's eat too many of the unhealthy and saturated fats. However, flax oil will help to put you into more of a "fatty acid balance."

Try 1 tablespoon per day.

7.) Glucosamine / Chondroitin

There is not research to support the fact that use of glucosamine/chondroitin will prevent the deterioration of joints, however it is logical to assume it does and may be a useful supplement ....considering the mounds of research that glucosamine/chondroitin does help slow the progression of osteoarthritis.

Recommended dose is 1500 mg glucosamine and 1200mg chondroitin per day.

8.) Food

No this really is not technically a supplement, however it's the most important component of any nutritional program..... so I had to mention it again.

Targeting your nutrients and timing your food intake really is the key.

DO NOT consider a dietary supplement until your nutrition program is solid. Once you are eating the whole grains, fruits, vegetables, lean proteins and healthy fats, then it may be time to consider supplements.

After the first few weeks have passed and we begin to implement supplements into the overall plan.......I recommend the more affordable and low dosage products.

If you are eating your diet, there will be no way you need 1000% of Vitamin C or 500% of Vitamin D and etc.
So spending a small fortune for expensive urine makes little to no sense at all.

I have put together a list of great quality, more than sufficient dosage and very affordable supplements at **Amazon.**

7. Your Successful Sleep Strategy

Sleep: Another Key to Fitness

How much thought do you put into the subject of "*how well you sleep*"?

How important do you think sleep really is to your Over-All success and performance?

What about your general health?

If you're like the majority of people, you probably don't think much about how "well" you sleep.

All people instinctively know they feel better when they sleep more, so it makes sense that you probably want to sleep well and tend to get unhappy when you don't sleep as much as you would like too.

But getting quality sleep is more than just about "sleeping a lot more". It also does a whole lot more for you than to make you feel a little bit better throughout the day. Quality sleep is actually one of the most important elements of your health, your workout program and your over-All performance and capabilities for improvement.

Like the science of nutrition and exercise, the science of sleep has been undergoing a new revolution over the last few decades.
Researchers are beginning to understand how sleep impacts our performance over the short term and long term.

Exactly how much can sleep impact you as an athlete?

Lets Consider the following:

• Researchers conducted a series of studies over a 30 year period.
National Football League game data demonstrated that teams which traveled between three time zones to play games at night experienced disrupted sleep and Exercise and diet schedules and were 67% more likely to lose..... even if the point spread was factored in.

• Studies show that athletes who consistently get roughly 10 hours of sleep per night show marked improvement in strength, speed, agility and reaction Time......... over the athletes performing on 8 or less hours.

• Athletes who get around 10 hours of sleep per night demonstrate a much better muscle memory for movements learned the day before.

• People not getting enough sleep are more prone to the effects of obesity, hypertension, diabetes and other various Cardio-metabolic and endocrine disorders.

• Research has shown that just a few days of little or no sleep impacts the body's insulin sensitivity by more than 25% in normal, healthy people. This essentially brings them into a pre-diabetic state— the equivalent of gaining 18 to 30 lb.

• Military research shows that sleep-deprived soldiers demonstrate a marked decrease in ability in marksmanship, judgment and the overall performance of mental and physical tasks.

• People who don't get enough sleep are often more Irritable, because a brain works differently when you are sleep deprived. An irritable athlete usually is not a very positive athlete.

Thus, sleep deprivation can rob you of your mental edge That is necessary for your success.

To see significant improvements in your performance, obviously you have to train properly and eat right. But without enough quality sleep, that work is nearly all wasted and could even be harmful for your body in the long term.

So behind and in a state so sleep deprived the body can't heal itself sufficiently.

Exercise, nutrition and sleep make a complete circle comprising the three essential elements of health and fitness.

You can't achieve your body's maximum potential in Over-All performance or be at peak levels of health, unless you pay attention and work hard toward focusing upon all elements.

Let's look a little deeper into the science behind why sleep is important to health and Over-All performance.

The Four Stages of your Sleep

Sleep occurs in cycles throughout the entire night, with each sleep cycle taking approximately 90 minutes. Your body's biological clock controls all of this stuff.

Technically speaking ....the sleep cycle is one of our many "circadian rhythms".

We have four identifiable stages in each of our sleep cycles; each has a significant impact on our Over-All performance and physical improvement.

- Stage one:

This lasts for about 20 minutes and this is the stage where your heart rate slows and your body temperature begins to cool down.

Your Brain activity during this time shows up in little "spindles," which are basically tightly packed brain-wave patterns. These spindles are linked to muscle memory and its "internalizing" of the movements you have learned during the daytime hours.

- Stage Two and Stage Three:

Stage Two is our transition from light sleep and into deep sleep.

Followed by Stage 3. Which is complete deep sleep when the body starts to produce very slow waves. This stage of sleep is often referred to as "slow-wave sleep," or SWS.

During this stage, our human growth hormone or HGH, is released and blood rushes from your brain to your muscles to begin to initiate recovery and reenergize the body.

Up to 70% of the body's daily production of HGH might occur during this state.

Additionally, elements of your "parasympathetic nervous system" are triggered while the "sympathetic nervous system" becomes suppressed.
All of this supports immune system function and your normal glucose metabolism during the day.

- Stage Four:

This stage is also known as "rapid-eye-movement sleep," or REM.

This is the stage where we have dreams.
Our arms and legs are completely paralyzed, and this is the only stage of your sleep where your body doesn't really move.

This stage of our sleep is associated with learning and memory retention, this is where the hippocampus transfers and then filters the day's information to your Neocortex.
This all works like a computer uploading information and then clearing its RAM onto a hard drive.

During the first few cycles, deep-sleep periods are longer and REM periods are shorter, but after the fourth cycle, REM periods start to become much longer and the deep-sleep phases much shorter.

The Important Benefits of your Slow-Wave Sleep:

• **Natural production of HGH**:
This is a particular hormone that the body naturally will produce. If we want to get stronger and faster, then we need our body to maximize natural production of HGH. You do this by getting adequate amounts of deep sleep. While it is true that most of our HGH released during the night is released in the first few of our sleep cycles.

• **Suppressing cortisol production**:
High levels of cortisol during the night create an insulin resistance in the morning, and it is linked to cardio-metabolic disorders ,such as, Type 2 diabetes and memory loss and cognitive impairment.

• **Suppression of your sympathetic nervous system in The favor of your parasympathetic nervous system**:

The sympathetic system is what is activated under stress, whereas the parasympathetic nervous system is what is activated by the body to recover and recuperate.

• **Release of prolactin**:

Has been shown to be correlated to proper immune system functioning.
Important Benefits of Stage 1 and REM stage Sleep Spindles are critical for the brain's ability to transfer learned muscle movements to the permanent memory. It is the period where your hippocampus transfers information to your neocortex, allowing you to recall the information, motor skills and other important information when you wake back up.
Without enough REM sleep, You can not remember and internalize important learned movements.

Athletes in sports that require highly skilled movements—like a snatch, clean and jerk, and Agility, where fractions of an inch are the difference between success and failure—need enough REM sleep to maintain and make improvements in performance.

Insufficient amounts of REM sleep will have a negative impact on the brain as a whole and causes it to function abnormally. As a consequence of this, the hippocampus works considerably less and other parts of the brain, such as the amygdala, are required to work more.

Because our amygdala is associated with rage and aggression, this would explain why sleep deprived people often are more irritable and moody.
Because a positive attitude is very important in sports, athletes simply can not afford any lapses that will cause them to lose their positive edge.

Sleeping for your Optimal Performance

You need to make a decision here and now to make sleep an integral part of your training program and that you are going to take it as seriously as your exercise and nutrition.

Block out at least nine hours of your day for sleep and ideally 10 hours of sleep. You might not actually sleep that long, but that should be your overall goal. We often fall short of what we set out to get done, so if you set out to get nine, you might just get eight, which is the required bare minimum for an athlete.

That said, everyone has very unique sleep needs, requirements and wants.
If you think you need nine and half hours of sleep a night to perform at a peak levels, then it is time to find that information out.

How would you know if you are sleeping enough? If you consistently wake up and feeling good without using an alarm clock....that is a strong sign that you are close to where you should to be in terms of sleep.

The Do's

- Eat better. Better nutrition helps with better sleep. In turn, sleep helps with metabolism. It's a never-ending cycle. To maximize the benefits of nutrition and sleep, you need to be doing both well.

- Give up on smoking or any other forms of tobacco.

- Perform Workouts late afternoon or early evening. Finish this workout before 7:30 pm. Our circadian rhythms prime our body for peak performance at this time of day. In contrast, early morning and late night are the circadian-rhythms low points for our performance. If you do multiple
workouts in a day, put the hardest one in the late afternoon or the early evening and avoid doing workouts too late or too early in the day.

- If doing a particularly hard set of workouts during the course of a week or month, be sure to get extra sleep during these stressful times to maximize your gains.

- Keep your room dark, quiet and cool while sleeping at night.
Light, hotter temperatures and excessive noise can disrupt Sleep patterns and will make you sleep poorly.

The Dont's

- Consume caffeine after the early afternoon. Caffeine can keep you up and shorten the length of time you sleep.

- Do not eat any big meals or have alcohol within 3 hours of going to bed. Particularly starchy carbohydrates

- Avoid taking long naps during the day.
Try to keep them under 90 minutes to avoid throwing off your biological clock. Long naps can have a similar effect on the body as jet lag. If you need to take a nap try to get in at least one full sleep cycle, or about 90 minutes, to avoid feeling groggy.

- Don't get up early just so you can do a workout and keep yourself from getting enough sleep. You are moving yourself backward, not forward. Your body needs sleep like it needs water or food.
You wouldn't deprive yourself of water so you could work out!
Because it would be very counterproductive.

- Do not watch anything that is on an electronic screen right before going to bed. Screens emit blue light, which essentially inhibits your production of melatonin and prevents you getting good sleep.

Sleep Systems

You spend more than one-third of your lifetime in bed, so dont you think that it might be worth it to get the right sleep system. Disruption of sleep, whether it be from "tossing and turning" or actually "waking up".....throws off your sleep patterns and deprives you of most of the true benefits of sleep.

Most people "wake up" and "toss and turn", because they sleep on an uncomfortable surface that cuts off circulation to their muscles during the night.

Here's what I recommend:

- A mattress that will create an airflow from top to bottom.

- Airflow keeps you cool while sleeping at night.

- A cool sleeping environment will help to sleep better and undisturbed.

- A mattress with softness and or firmness that you can Customize and control.

- A pillow that is as soft or firm and thick or thin as you like it to be.

Sleep Well, Train Hard

At this point you probably are worrying that **you** are not reaching your full potential, simply because you're not sleeping enough.

That's actually a good thing, because it's likely true.

It is simply a matter of keeping in mind that sleeping better isn't very difficult; it just takes some effort and discipline on your part.

Yeah, I know...... 10 hours sounds like a lot of sleep.
So just Trust me as a coach. As an athlete you probably need more sleep if you want to maximize any of your hard earned gains or progress in any significant manner.

The best news/secret in this manual is that THIS dumb little tidbit is usually the easiest way to see significant improvements in over-all health and performance.

So by just following some of the above information, you should be well on your way to better health and much better fitness levels.

In Summary

Try to fit a few 90-minute naps into your schedule during the week.

Even if its just 2 or 3 days a week.

I cant stress enough how much this one aspect can increase performance.

Adjust this one key ingredient and see huge gains.

Especially when just beginning this new program.

8. Your balance and flexibility

Stretching and Flexibility

Slow Stretching

If you are involved in any form of fitness or physical training, and particularly in traditional sports, you already have been using the "slow static" stretching regiments for years. This form of stretching is okay and can be very conducive when performed at the right times and in the proper amounts.

I have given a few reasons why excessive amounts of static or passive stretching can actually be counter-productive while you are training for an improvement in sports performance :   *{Listen-up my Yoga Junkies}*

- Relaxing of your nervous system, which causes decreased neural firing
- Mild fatigue
- Decreased coordination
- Decrease in agility
- Decrease in quickness
- Weakens the stretch reflex

All of the above side-effects are brought on by the **"relaxation"** of the nervous system which is responsible for all your different movements.

As can be see from the list, if the nervous system gets too relaxed, there will be no way you will perform at an optimal performance level.

Having your Static stretches performed **post** workout can offer the trainee the best of all benefits ,such as, a mental relaxation, calming of the nervous system and your static flexibility.

An Enhanced overall recovery time is another nice benefit.

Dynamic Range Of Motion Stretching

"Dynamic Range of Motion" stretching is exactly what we need **before** intense exercise. The following are a few benefits and the advantages that can be expected with the use of a proper Range of Motion program:

- Increased neural firing
- Coordination
- Stability
- Muscle lengthening
- Heightened body awareness
- Balance
- Improved agility and quickness

As you can obviously see all of these qualities are just what any athlete, performer or average Joe would want to acquire and have.

These are the qualities that make the difference between an average Joe and a super-star.

Isometric Stretching

"Isometric stretching" uses positions similar to those used with "Static passive", but adding some strong tensions of the muscles which are being stretched. The benefits of this particular type of stretching will be particularly important for gymnasts or grapplers or etc.

Static holds are performed with weights and can improve overall flexibility greatly. When executing static holds with weights simply hold a weight at a particular angle that stretches the intended muscle and joint sufficiently.

An example of this form of stretching would be to sit at the bottom of a front squat while holding a weight for designated time period.

Be very cautious and careful when using these techniques though.

Effects On Performance

All of the stretches mentioned above can have many positive effects upon your performance in your specific sport.

Having an adequate flexibility or your ability to move your joints through their entire intended full range, without there becoming a decrease in your absolute strength.

This is required for you to perform at your top optimal levels.

As previously stated, it is also quite important that you have an understanding of what types of flexibility are most needed for their sport or activity.

Do not forget that the manner in which a trainee performs his/her sport should also be taken into consideration when developing his or her personal stretching and flexibility program.

For example, If you are someone who likes throwing high kicks, quick jumps or likes to pull off wide splits...... Then having more hip mobility should be one top priority.

If, in this instance, you are a Fitness Model on her/his feet 10 hours before a crowd of thousands.....this attribute would not be as significant and therefore attention would be focused elsewhere.

Flexibility

Flexibility can be defined as:

"the absolute range of movement in a joint or series of joints that is attainable in a momentary effort."

From this definition we can deduce that flexibility is not something very "general" at all. It is very specific to a particular joint or set of joints within the body.

It is a complete myth that some people are naturally more flexible throughout their total body. Just being extremely flexible in one certain location or joint does not necessarily guarantee your being flexible in another area. Being "limber" in the upper body does not mean you will automatically be "limber" in your lower body.

According to Researchers, flexibility in a joint is also specific to the action performed and the requirements of that joint.

Having the ability to do a front-splits does not imply the ability to do a side-splits, even though both actions occur at the same exact hip.

Different Types of Flexibility

Many people are not even aware of the fact that there are different types of flexibility. The several different flexibility types are categorized according to the various types of activities involved in athletic training and performance.

The flexibilities which involve some type of motion are called "dynamic" and the ones which do not involve motion are called "static".

The different types of flexibility are:

Dynamic flexibility

Dynamic flexibility , which is also referred to as your "kinetic flexibilities", equals the ability to perform dynamic movements of the muscles to bring a limb through its full range of motion in and at the joints.

Static-active flexibility

Static-active flexibility , can also be referred to as your "active flexibilities", and it is the ability that you acquire and then fully maintain an extended position using only the tension of the agonists and synergists while the antagonists are being stretched-out. For example... while lifting your leg and keeping it high without any outside support ,except from ONLY your own leg muscles.

Static-passive flexibility
Static-passive flexibility , also referred to as "passive flexibilities", is the ability that you can acquire and then fully maintain extended positions and then maintain them using only your own weight, the support of your limbs, or with some other apparatus ....such as a chair or a bar.

Note also that the ability to maintain this position does not come solely from your muscles alone, like it does with the static-active flexibility. The ability to do a full-splits would be an example of your static-passive flexibility.

Research has shown that active flexibility is very closely associated to levels of sports achievement than is passive flexibility. Active flexibilities are more difficult to develop and achieve than your passive flexibilities ,which is what the average person thinks of as "flexibility".

Not only does your "active flexibility" require "passive flexibility" in order to assume any initial extended positions, But it does also require you to have the muscle strength to be able to hold and maintain those positions.

Strength training and flexibility training should both go along together. It is a quite common misconception that there must always be a trade-off between your flexibility and your strength.

Certainly, if you ignore your flexibility training altogether in order to train for strength then you are certainly sacrificing your overall flexibility and obviously vice versa.

Performing and training for both strength and flexibility need not sacrifice either over the other.

Your flexibility and your strength training will actually enhance one another quite nicely.

Putting it all together

One of the best times to stretch is right after a workout, such as lifting weights, swimming or sparring. Static stretching of fatigued and tired muscles are performed immediately following the workout that caused the fatigue.

This helps not only to increase your flexibility, but it also helps to enhance the promotion of your muscular development. It will also literally decrease the level of your post-workout soreness.

Here's why:

After you have stressed, overloaded and fatigued a particular muscle.....
that muscle retains a certain "pump" and it becomes somewhat shortened.
This "shortening" is due mostly in part to the repetition of intense muscle activity that often only takes the muscle through part of its full range of motion.

The "pump" makes the muscle appear larger. A "pumped-up" muscle is also very full of lactic acid and other by-products from the intense activity. If stretching of the muscle is not done after a workout, it will kind of "retain" the decreased range of motion ,as it "forgets" how to make itself as long as it could be again, and with the buildup of the lactic acid will cause you to experience postexercise soreness.

Static stretching of your "pumped-up" muscle will help it to become considerably "looser", and to once again "remember" its full range of movement.

This also helps in the removal of lactic acid and other waste-products. It is true that stretching a "pumped-up" muscle will make it appear visibly smaller to the naked eye, but it does not decrease the muscle's actual size at all ,nor will it inhibit the muscle growth.
It merely reduces the "Tightness" ,also known as contraction, which is merely a reduced state of your muscles so that they do not have that "bulge" quite as much.

Also, strenuous and intense workouts will often cause damage to the connective tissues of the muscle. These connective tissues heal in roughly 1 to 2 days, but it is also believed that these connective tissues will heal at a shorter length and will therefore decreasing muscular development
and your flexibility at the same time.

In order to prevent this tissue from healing with the shorter lengths, physiologists, coaches and trainers recommend using "static stretching" **after** your strenuous workouts.

On a final note , Flexibility equals one of the easiest motor qualities an athlete can attain and develop with just a little time and practice, no matter what your fitness or talent level.

In terms of "Flexibility", DNA or genetics have no limit upon your ability to attain this quality.

This means prioritizing this quality appropriately and training at it with a great focus.

Spending 3 minutes per day "Static" stretching before you workout will do little to enhance this important quality.

9. Your Speed and Agility

Agility

For our purposes, Agility can be defined as the ability to start explosively, decelerate immediately, then quickly change direction and then accelerate up again very quickly and efficiently ....all while maintaining your body control and minimizing any drop in speed.

Agility can often be defined as an athlete's combined coordination of abilities. These are all the elements of your basic technical skills that are used to perform motor tasks spanning the power spectrum from dynamic activities to fine motor control tasks and including ability to adapt, combine abilities, balance, accurate orientation, reactiveness, differentiation and overall rhythm.

"Coordinative abilities" are often recognized to be most easily developed in preadolescence and teen years, which is considered to be an important time period for skill development.

This period often changes focus during young adult period, when the shift from general to special preparation usually begins.

Most sports activities that utilize "Agility" occur in 10 seconds or less and involve the ability to coordinate several "sport specific" tasks simultaneously, such as catching a football and then making a series of evasive moves and cuts to avoid being tackled in order to advance the ball further down the field.

With the exception of skills sets that are specific to a particular sport, Agility can be the primary determining factor to predict success in a sport or fitness activity.

Typically all Sports require changes of direction in which lateral movements are used in the several planes of movement simultaneously. Sports are regularly played in short bursts of under 30 feet (10 yards) before a change of direction, acceleration or deceleration is required.

Because movements can begin from various body alignments and centers, Athletes and Trainees need to be able to react with strength, explosiveness and quickness from these several different positions.

Some people in athletics may believe that Agility is primarily determined by genetic makeup and is therefore difficult or impossible to improve or enhance to any significant level.

Sports Coaches & Trainers often become enamored with an athlete that possesses natural physical attributes such as: actual size, vertical &/or horizontal power, ideal body, strength...... that are generally associated with a successful performance in certain sport.

However, many Coaches and Trainers often find these attributes alone will not guarantee success in any particular sport that requires Agility.

Unfortunately, because of the focus placed on physical attributes, the focus on your "off-season" programs often revolves around strength training and conditioning.

Often an athletes Agility ,as well as, speed development at sport-specific speeds are forgotten, neglected or only focused upon during tiny blocks of time in the "pre-season".

Agility is a neural/natural ability that is developed over time with many thousands of repetitions. The nervous system, its motor abilities and sport specific movements at sport-specific speeds will have little time for advancement ,let alone development, if not addressed during the "off-season".

It takes Athletes or Trainees weeks and months of attention to see any improvements in speed and Agility. Agility should be trained as a very important component of your annual and on-going training program.

Athletes and/or Trainees who train for power-oriented sports by only strength training and not incorporating sport-specific Agility training are making a huge mistake in reaching their absolute best performance enhancement for their chosen sport.

Whether it is a basketball player cutting toward a pass, a football lineman pulling to trap a defensive lineman or an MMA fighter, Agility is a crucial and often overlooked component of athletic performance.

In sports such as baseball or Cheer.... lateral speed Agility and quickness can be just as essential as strength and speed.

The performances of Athletes and Trainees in sports today have dramatically elevated the level of Agility necessary to performance and success.

There is a direct correlation between improved Agility and the development of athletic abilities such as : coordination, rhythm, timing, and movement.

The key to improving Agility is to minimize a loss of speed while redirecting your body's center of gravity.

Drills requiring rapid changes of movement such as, forward- backward, vertically- laterally and will help you improve your Agility ,as well as, your coordination by training your body to make these changes in movement more quickly and efficiently.

The Performance Benefits of "Agility Training"

Sports Coaches & Trainers may have some difficulty at bridging the gap between applied use of strength, power and cardio conditioning developed in conjunction with strength training and conditioning for a particular activity or sport.

Even for the athlete who will never become that Mega-Super-Star who shake the planet and bring the viewing audience to its feet..........
Agility training has many critical benefits that an athlete can receive through Agility training.

1.) Neuro-muscular Adaptation:

Agility training may be the most effective way to address the neuro-muscular system and sport-specific skills necessary for improving your sport performance; Since Agility training most closely resembles that of the activity itself.

Training using sport-specific metabolic training speeds enables Athletes and Trainees to train at a level that most closely resembles the intensity, duration, and recovery time found in their particular sport , while training during the off-season.

The use of Agility training in an annual training program provides a critical link for Athletes or Trainees to apply their strength and conditioning program gains to the competitive athletic arena.

2.) Improvements in Athleticism:

The most critical benefit of Agility training is increased body control resulting from a concentrated form of overall body awareness. Athletes and Trainees that begin to effectively incorporate a consistent Agility program into their overall training, often talk of the stunning gains in athleticism; actual sport played didn't matter!

It teaches the intricacies of controlling small transitions around the neck, in the shoulders, back, hips, the knees and ankle joints for the best posture alignment.

Athletes and Trainees gain a sense of control over the task of moving faster. This can be seen in a greater overall sense for the uncoordinated athlete who learns more about him or herself through Agility training than the already coordinated athlete.

3.) Injury Prevention and a Decrease in Rehabilitation Time:

While it is virtually impossible to eliminate injury as whole; Agility training will improve your "Athletic Injury Management system".

Injuries are definitely not just a result of an athlete having bad luck.
By possessing the ability to control your body during that split second or critical moment of impact, a possible injury can often be prevented or its severity reduced considerably. This requires preparing the body for the strange, unbalanced and unfamiliar movements, which can occur in sports and may result in an injury.

By using activity-specific movements that imitate your activity under low to moderate stress and speed levels in practice situations and through Agility training, an athlete's body becomes more prepared for specific movements and therefore injuries can be prevented and/or greatly reduced.

When Athletes and Trainees utilize Agility drills, they develop that neuro-muscular awareness and thus are better able to understand the movements of their own bodies.

Any rehabilitation process can then move much more rapidly if the injured athlete possesses such neurological awareness and flexibility.

Components of an Agility Training program

A comprehensive Agility program will address the following components of Agility itself: the strength component, overall power, acceleration & deceleration, combined coordination with balance and dynamic flexibility.

When formulating an Agility program for athletic performance enhancement, a Coach or Trainee should incorporate the following components of Agility:

1.) Strength – Strength refers to a maximal force that a particular muscle or muscle group can generate at a specified velocity or distance & time.

When an athlete is in contact with an opponent, the addition of the opponent's resistance *plus* your own body weight is the total of resistance.

A lot of research has determined a strong correlation between lower body strength and Agility.

The more emphasis the sport has on strength and power the greater the need for strength training, particularly the "Olympic lifts" area, and importantly where the rate of your force development is most similar to that of Agility movements of the specific sport you perform.

In my "On-Season/Competition season program", I like to switch those "Olympic Lifts" to a lot of Volume Training with bodyweight-ish weights and I add a few Agility-type lifts (IE: Walking Barbell Lunges).

Getting my Athletes and Trainees ready to easily and most efficiently move their opponents bodyweight around.

2.) Power – Power is a rate at which work is completed or force *times* velocity. The faster an athlete gets from point A to point B....the greater his/her power.

3.) Acceleration – Acceleration is any change in velocity per a designated unit of time. It is an athlete's ability to go from a starting position to a greater velocity and then change from one speed to another.
In the sport of Triathlon, they call it "Shifting Gears".

4.) Deceleration – Deceleration is recognized as an ability to decrease speed or stop from a maximal or near maximal speed.
Deceleration can be performed in various forms from using single or multiple footsteps, backpedaling, shuffling, or using a crossover step to slow down or come to a complete stop.

5.) Coordination – Coordination is defined as an ability to control and process muscle movements to produce the most efficient athletic skills or abilities.

6.) Dynamic Balance – Dynamic balance is the ability to maintain control over your body while in motion. When your body is in motion, various feedback from the body, such as sight, awareness and equilibrium are made by the nervous system to adjust the center of gravity.

It's a fact that Agility is closely aligned with balance by requiring Athletes and Trainees to regulate shifts in the body's center of gravity, while subjecting them to adjustments in posture.

7.) Dynamic Flexibility – Dynamic flexibility is the range of motion at a body's joint during active times of movement. These are mostly activities utilized as a part of your warm-up and are designed to increase flexibility, sharpens coordination, increases speed and aligns balance.
Also known as "Stretching out".

Technique

When instructing Trainees on the execution of "Agility exercises", I find it is crucial to instruct them on technique.

Visual focus, arm action and reaction, deceleration, recovery and particular biomechanics all play a valuable role in the proper technique of your "Agility drills".

1.) Visual Focus – The athlete's head should always be in a neutral position with eyes focused directly forward, regardless of the direction or movement pattern being used by the athlete.

Obviously certain exceptions to this guideline will occur when the athlete is required to focus on another athlete or object during training.

Additionally, getting the head around and finding a new focus point should initiate all directional changes and transitions.

2.) Arm Action – Powerful arm movements during transitional and directional changes is critical in order to acquire a higher speeds.
Use of inadequate or improper arm movement may result in a loss of speed or efficiency.

3.) Deceleration – The ability of an athlete to decelerate from a given velocity is going to be crucial for the athlete in changing directions.

4.) Recovery – When training Athletes to enhance their Agility it is important to ensure that drills are performed at work and rest intervals consistent with the sport the athlete is training for.

Partner Athletes with other Athletes of similar abilities. They Perform drills and exercises in a competitive atmosphere with technique always being more critical than the speed the drill is performed.

5.) Biomechanics – When it comes to training for biomechanics and "Agility training", three overlapping or correlating considerations should be taken :

A.) Body Alignment – Maintaining your lower center of gravity enables the athlete to move considerably quicker and with increased decelerate and reaccelerate; especially when requiring the overcoming of the resistance of an opponent or an object.

The maintenance of a core stability (or the maintaining a neutral spine throughout the exercise) and the athletic position .....or perfect posture with the shoulders pulled back and down and tighten the abdominals, with knees slightly bent and with hips back and down.

Your full bodyweight forward on the middle of your feet ,will enable the athlete to supply and train to provide maximum power.

B.) Movement Economy – Athletes and Trainees need to be educated as to the most efficient movement and patterns and to develop the required skills necessary to reach their individual goals.

The certain patterns and skills may include movement patterns or skills that include side shuttling, backsprinting, use of a cross stepping, get-up, turn and run or combinations of these patterns and skills.

C.) Acceleration & Deceleration – Most sports require Athletes and Trainees to have the ability to accelerate, then decelerate and then reaccelerate again.

The more efficient an athlete becomes at this the better the athlete becomes at creating space between an opponent, and the more able to move more quickly to a space or object and enhance performance potential.

Outside of an athletes already attained sport specific experience and/or training, Agility training may end up becoming the primary determining factor to predict success for an athlete in a sport.

Activities usually are not performed "straight ahead" and typically require changes of direction in which lateral movements are used in several planes of movement at the same time.

Since movements in sport are initiated from multiple and various body positions, Athletes and Trainees need to be able to react with strength, explosiveness and quickness from all of these varying positions.

Because of the focus placed primarily upon genetic physical attributes in sports, most of the focus on off-season programs often revolves around strength training exclusively.

As stated before, Agility and speed development at your sport-specific speeds are usually neglected and/or only focused upon during small blocks of time in the pre-season. Agility is a nervous systems ability that is developed over time with hundreds of repetitions.

Research shows that an increase in speed and strength was not nearly as effective in developing Agility as participation in activities specifically designed to develop Agility.

Training for increased Agility

As we have covered, Agility can be defined as the ability to accelerate quickly, decelerate immediately and rapidly change the body direction while maintaining control and balance.

The key element in Agility training to expose the athlete to a vast array of different movement patterns and drills. Agility training should be treated as a training of your Nervous System and NOT a big endurance training event. The nervous system needs to be somewhat "Limber" to maximize its ability to learn.

My Athletes and Trainees perform Agility training anywhere from 1-4 times per week. Usually as a warm-up to a big endurance event. This usually depends on the individual athlete and his or her specific sport.

If an individual shows fantastic movement in his or her sport already, minimal time is needed to be spent training this quality.

On the other hand if the guy cannot box without falling over his feet , then a considerable amount of time is spent working on his ability to move.
There are some authorities in this industry that claim the only way to enhance sport specific Agility is by performing the sport. I would not agree with this.

As an example boxing requires several separate "motor qualities". By training the qualities each separately, there is a more concentrated effort on each of those particular qualities.

There are numerous research studies and practical case studies that have and will support this statement.

Quickness Drills

Quickness training is another skill set usually neglected by Athletes and Trainees and their coaches.
This includes coaches in about every sport .

It amazes me whenever I meet an athlete that has spent Years, Months, days and hours performing sprints and ridiculously useless training exercises all while over training.... yet does absolutely no Agility or quickness training. If he does, its by accident from some ancient Chinese martial art technique or Hollywood Movie/Rocky tactic that usually has no place in an actual sport.

In most sports or daily activities, there is a need for constant change of direction and Reacting to ever changing situations.

Quickness =
A Rapid reaction time and counter movement in response to a given stimuli.

Keep in mind there is an overlapping between Agility and "Quickness training"; as several drills will promote both of these particular qualities.
Quickness can be thought of as a *unit of speed*.

Speed as it relates to specific activities particularly refers to a measurement of distance reached in a specified amount of time.

Speed of movement is a function of a combination of quickness, reactive-ability, endurance, strength, and skill. The ability to coordinate one's movements in response to many external conditions under which the motor task is to be executed.

An athlete can possess good speed while at the same time still be lacking in quickness.

An example would be an athlete who punches a speed bag with quick hands, but then appears to be slow when throwing punches while sparring or fighting. This is usually a case of slow reaction time and a tight and non-relaxed body.

In a training program to enhance an athletes quickness, I prescribe a variety of drills into my programs. These drills include reactionary drills, quick hands and quick feet exercises. The main emphasis is an instant reaction and movement to a given stimulus.

The drills are usually quite short in duration ,usually 6-8 seconds. The majority of the time quickness drills are performed before strength training or cardio training. If the goal is to improve "quickness endurance", they will be performed after the strength training session for 10-16 seconds.

This rehearsal helps to reinforce the qualities associated with that of being fatigued at the end of the game or bout and still being able to execute quick movements. A good base of general quickness is established before moving onto quickness endurance drills; which are a more advanced skillset designed to build upon general quickness. The frequency of quickness training varies accordingly.

Athletic Movement-Type Agility Training Sessions

These agility runs are designed as interval training where you will perform a specific sprint and/or change of direction run followed up by a slow jog or walk as an active rest back to your starting point.

These types of runs are perfect for most sports that involve a variety of movement patterns during performance. These types of runs are effective because of the specific type of training.... meaning most sports do not only involve straight ahead running.

For example, soccer, lacrosse, Cheer, softball, baseball, & football all require bouts of high intensity running or work and recovery bouts such as slow jogging, walking, or resting in place.

Each run should be performed at 100% of your intensity.
Have a starting point on your training surface. After each sprint, jog back at a recovery pace to your starting point and then perform the next sprint.

A 1:3 work to rest ratio is perfect. This means you will work the sprint and then recover 3x's longer than the sprint time (i.e. sprint :10 = recover :30).
Make sure you always get a very good warm-up in so your body is prepared for this type of intense sport specific interval workout.

This training can be done in almost any setting.

A field, gym, court, parking lot, really any open space can be utilized to train. You may have to modify some of the distances, but the important thing is that you must work at 100% of your intensity to really utilize these change of direction runs.

This is where you take the strength from the weight room, your strength program, and apply it to your athletic arena where it really matters.

Strength training will enhance your overall strength and speed for your sport, now you must apply that through sport specific running and drilling programs.

You may perform these types of training sessions
2-3 times per week (3 times per week pre-season).

These runs are ideal training for a pre-season athlete. Base the number of sprints on your conditioning level and how your body feels.

A speed training session should not be longer than **1.5 to 2 miles** or **20-30 minutes** and you may also use your heart rate monitor as a guideline for intensity.

Brining it all together

The general goal of our agility training here at the foundation level is to do just that.....build a base of exercises and a foundation of agility skills and abilities from which to advance and build upon.

We want to know what you can and cant do and then begin to put them into use on a regular basis.

10. Your Strength and Conditioning

Strength Training and Conditioning Program

What we are going to cover in this section:

1. Learn how to properly perform weight training exercises that transform Your Body.

2. Learn our Base Strength Training Program.

3. Get yourself an exercise journal put together.

4. Learn how to record your data properly from each workout.

5. Learn how to interpret all of the data to transform your body.

6. Plan your training times during the day & week so you will never miss workouts.

7. Get in the Gym and Go Hard.

Once we have your Nutritional Program all calculated and dialed-in, the next factor required is to transform your body through the use of a proper training program. There are a lot of training secrets in this program to ensure you get lean and built like nothing you've ever been before.

This program has been assembled not just from theory, but from good old hard work transforming many many athletes and clients over more than two decades.
It works. And in some cases when nothing else has or will.

My program does and will assume that you know all of the standard exercises for weight/resistance training.
This course is not about having to re-write the thousands upon thousands of works on the subject of " health and fitness ".
It is designed to be the guidelines of a year long program. A program designed to teach you about you, while using all the above mentioned research.

A "Condensed" version of EVERYTHING you need to know

Here is a crash course on some of the raw basics for you to get the most out of your Workouts and training sessions.

Is it true that you are just going to the gym to hoist around weights?
Yes..... the more you lift the bigger ,leaner and more efficient your muscles will grow; but it is not exactly that simple.

Lifting too much for your current condition and goal can lead to overtraining and no gains or improvement at all. There's probably a good chance this has already happened to you at some point.

When you are training, you need to consistently push yourself "strategically" to allow your body to adapt to the daily/weekly increasing stress you are placing on it.

Stress upon muscles (Weight lifting)
+   = GROWTH
Recovery (Nutrition & Rest)

This flow chart seems pretty simple and it is. What makes transforming your body into an amazing growth and performance spike so tricky.....
is the fact that every person is different.

No two people respond the same way to weight training or recover at the same exact rates. The whole secret to really exploding muscle growth and fat loss is to figure out your recovery and training frequency ratio.

Most programs and trainers will simply prescribe a pre-set structure which does not change, but remains the same regardless of your current fitness level.
The same workouts his other clients do.
This is the reason why most athletes fail at achieving their dreams.

That is why this program is designed to teach YOU to eventually become your own "Personal Trainer/Coach" and your own "Dietitian".

Your muscles must be fully recovered from your previous workout or training session in order to make your best forward progress.

The amount of time required for you to fully recover increases as does your ability to train more intensely and with heavier weights.

So as you continue to get stronger, you will need to figure out how to stress your muscles continually harder to keep continually growing.

As you train your muscles harder and harder, you will require more and more recovery time as well.

In other words, as you increase your training intensity and your training weight .....you need to increase your recovery time.

At some certain point, the amount of rest required to recover will not be any greater for you..... no matter how heavy and intense you train.

Our Basic Structure

There are two terms you need to know to understand this program, a "phase" and a "cycle". Once you do you can unleash the power of amazing progress.

This "Four Phase" program is a daily routine made up of several different and unique training routines. Each training routine equals a training "phase".

Each "phase" has its specific focus and is specifically designed to work with the other "phase" creating a synergistic and systematic training growth effect.

A "cycle" is the time it takes to complete each "phase".
We have three different "cycles" : begin, intermediate and advanced.

The number of "cycles" basically determines the number of times you workout or train per week.

Start with workouts in the "beginner training cycle" and stick to it until according to your recuperation and recovery needs and progressive increases in power......it's probably time to advance to the next training "cycle".

Training "phases" are completed every time you complete one training "cycle". So when one training "Cycle" is finished, then you start the next type of training "phase".

For example. As a beginner you will train on the schedule determined by the "beginner training cycle". You will start with the training "phase one". So you go to the charts and see that this means that you will train three times per week. Possibly every second day and finish off the "cycle" in four
weeks time.

As soon as one of the "cycles" is completed, you start another "cycle" of training.....now you are onto training "phase two". After you have gone through four different training "phases"....compare your gathered data from your charts.

If all factors increased by at least 3 percent then continue with training "cycle one".

If your data factors do not continue to increase...... then that is probably your signal to start training at the next cycle level.
At the outset it is highly likely you will have very large percentage increases (20 – 50%) in your overall performance. As you become more advanced it is likely You will see considerably smaller, but consistent increases and gains.
This is considered normal.

As you become stronger and stronger, it is much harder to push your limits more and more. A slight advance becomes much to brag about. Once you are not making smaller and smaller advances.......
then it is time to move up to a more advanced training cycle.

So to summarize everything so far...... stick to the same training "cycle" and only progress to the next training "cycle" as determined by your power increases.

If your power increases start to level off or stop altogether (3% or less); then it is time to go to the next training "cycle".

Training "phases" rotate at the completion of every training "cycle".

A "cycle" basically is a *cycle* of each training "phase".

I hope this is explained thoroughly because it is a very precise scientific method of monitoring progress...yet it is not that complex once you get to it.

How we adjust recovery time

So we can gauge the time you need to recover accurately a method of measuring the intensity and work completed by each muscle is required. Almost no other program of training has this level of mathematically and scientifically adjusting recovery time.

Let's review some things, so we can accurately measure our muscular output.

There are three units of measure for each set:

1. Number of repetitions

2. Number of sets

3. Time set is completed measured in seconds/minutes from start to finish of the exercise

Use this data to figure out the power-factor.

A power-factor is an easy calculation adapted from physics.

What it figures out is the amount of work done per minute.......
And is measured in a pounds per minute (lbs/min) equation.

The exercise journal provided is designed to conveniently record each measurement for each workout.

Let's take a look at how to use the data that you record from each workout. For our example here, the Bench Press will be used.

Exercise	Set #	#Repetitions	weight	Time	Power
Bench Press	1	10	200	½ min	4000 lbs/min
Bench Press	2	1	315	10 sec	1890 lbs/min

Using the above chart...... the Power is calculated as follows:

(Number of repetitions) X (Weight Used) = POWER (lbs/ min) Time in minutes

Add the power number for each set together and get your total per body part. Add all your combined totals per workout to get a total per workout.

Record your power by doing the following workout every 8 weeks.

- Squats

- Bench press

- Dead Lift

- Overhead press

The goal here is to always consistently be increasing your power-factor every eight weeks by a few Percent points. If you are a beginner your power-factor will increase quite rapidly for the first few months of your training.

As you become more and more advanced the more the effort and new methods will be required to make significant gains.

Your power-factor will make increases from the following:

- Increasing training weights lifted while completing the same amount of sets and reps in the same amount of time.

- Increasing the amount of completed repetitions performed in a set period of time and number of sets.

- By performing fixed weight repetitions and sets, only doing it in less amount of time.

(The formula does not apply to "Rest Pause" types of training or my SuperSlow principle of training. }

Time is increased as a means to increasing the training intensity.
What a rip off it would be, if you held a heavy weight for a longer period of time, but when you calculated your power-factor the pounds per minute were less. Right?

It requires very complex mathematics and physics to make accurate "guesses" for these types of calculations. Its nearly impossible to calculate an individual's effort relative to the work being performed.

There are too many variables in your human anatomy from person to person that make even attempting to create an accurate universal-type formula not worth the effort for the extra benefit it would provide.

For this reason, it is our goal here to make gauging progress as practical as possible for the purpose of making any leaps in progress. For this reason we stick to measuring the recommended exercises and only under the prescribed strict time conditions.

For example; when measuring your power-factor on the bench press, keep your effort similar to all of your previous efforts......Probably a consistent speed that is pretty slow if you are using heavy weight.

Time to complete the test set should ideally be quite close to the time taken to finish the set you are trying to beat previously. Focus on increasing the number of repetitions completed with greater training poundages.

When training to transform your body, optimal recovery is needed to support optimum training conditions and optimal forward progress.

How we Recover Between Workouts for optimal Results

To make an optimal recovery between your workouts the following formulas must be in place:

1. Lots of nutrients at all times in the bloodstream to support muscle repair & growth.

2. A lot of quality sleep and rest

3. Handle life stress properly

4. Having a healthy body including kidneys, heart, lungs, liver and joints

5. Optimal hormone production

6. Enough time between workouts to fully recuperate for another workout

Considering items one through five are all in order of importance, our goal then, is to properly adjust the time between workouts to sustain a maximum efficiency.

For optimum results, it is assumed that the more you train .....as in your overall experience and not length of your actual workouts.....the more effective you will be at increasing your intensity.

As you increase your intensity more , more rest is required.

This workout program has three rest "cycles".

The first "cycle" has considerably less recuperation time and far more frequent workouts. As your training progresses, the training frequency gets to be less.

For example, instead of training every second day, as we do in the first "cycle". The second "cycle" you will now be training every third day.

As you can see, an extra recuperation day between training sessions is added as you become more advanced. As you are able to train more and with greater and greater intensity , you put more and more stress on the body.

The extra rest time between workouts helps:

** Keep Cortisol levels as low as humanly possible, to allow your natural anabolic hormones to have their greatest growth effects.

** Giving liver and kidneys the proper time to recuperate.

** Decreases constant the strain on tendons and ligaments from heavy lifting and training.

** Gives muscles a lot of time to recuperate and repair.

Following are samples of training schedules with rest days laid out:

Cycle One

Monday	Tuesday	Wed	Thursday	Friday	Sat	Sunday
Workout1	Rest	Workout2	Rest	Workout3	Rest	Rest
Workout1	Rest	Workout 2	Rest	Workout3	Rest	Rest

Cycle Two

Monday	Tuesday	Wednesday	Thursday	Friday	Saturday	Sunday
Workout1	Rest	Rest	Workout2	Rest	Rest	Workout3
Workout1	Rest	Workout2	Rest	Rest	Workout3	Rest

Cycle Three

Monday	Tuesday	Wednesday	Thursday	Friday	Sat	Sunday
Workout1	Rest	Rest	Rest	Workout2	Rest	Rest
Rest	Workout3	Rest	Rest	Rest	Workout1	Rest
Rest	Rest	Workout 2	Rest	Rest	Rest	Workout3

Knowing Exactly When It's Time to Get More Rest and Recuperation

Monitoring your progress and knowing when to advance to the next training "cycle", Will be monitoring your power calculations for your test exercises once per every 8 weeks.

Besides the actual power calculations, compare your increases in power from week to week.

As soon as a plateauing or tapering-off of any gradual but constant progress in power occurs.... it is then time to move to the next training frequency "cycle".

For example, if you currently train in "cycle" one. You find that you regularly make increases in power of 10- 12 percent every training "phase".

Now.... after calculating your *current* power-factor, you see a less than a 5 percent increase in power was made this phase.

BINGO! This is your scientific means of measurement!

THIS is your signal to advance to training "cycle" number 2.

Once you arrive in training "cycle" three, rarely will more rest help to increase progress.

Remember our goal is to transform your body into an efficient machine, not just get stronger.

When training plateaus occur during this cycle, try some of the following techniques to break plateaus:

1. Switch to the volume training plan for two weeks.

2. Take a full week or two off from training. (drills / cardio= Recommended instead)

3. Increasing your caloric intake by a few hundred calories per day for awhile.

4. Cut out or back on cardio.

5. Increase total sleep time.

The techniques above assume that all these factors are already at optimal.

Keep in mind that every person is going to progress at quite different rates.
Some people may gradually increase in power by four or five percent every four "phases" rather consistently.

A drop of a percent or two is enough information to consider more rest.
For other subjects a usual power-factor increase of 10 percent may be normal.

For these people a drop to 5 percent is a good signal to move on to the next training "cycle".

For all subjects..... more experience will result in your power-factor increasing more gradually over time.

As you become more experienced do not become discouraged by smaller percentage increments, this is the constant.

How to Figure Out a power-factor Percentage Increase

To figure out the percentage increase of your power-factor, we use the following equation:

You will need your prior power-factor which we will refer to as -
Old Number

And your new power-factor calculation which we will refer to as -
New Number

Your New Number minus the Old Number = Difference In lbs/min

Difference Divided by Old Number and Multiplied by 100 =

Percentage Increase in Power (Difference of Old power-factor X 100)

Monitor your percentage of increases and use it to know exactly how much and when to proceed to your next training frequency "cycles".

Training Methods

This is a guide to the various training methods recommended for accelerated progress accompanied by a thorough explanation of each method.

Drop Sets

Drop Sets are executed by beginning your exercise set with your maximum three to five repetition weight, doing as many repetitions as possible(2-6) then immediately dropping your exercise weight to exactly seventy percent of the weight you were just using and doing as many repetitions as
possible.

This process is repeated again with fifty percent of your first set weight then once more with thirty percent to really finish off the body part you are working.....Or it is performed as a set prescribed amount of drop increments; As it relates to sports specific movements.

If you can do more than two of these drop sets it is not because you are strong. On the contrary ,it is because you are not pushing yourself hard enough.

An example for Dumbbell chest Press follows:

- Begin with 100 pound dumbbells for the first set of four to six repetitions.

- Immediately do as many reps as possible with seventy pounds.

- Immediately do as many reps as possible with fifty pound dumbbells.

- Immediately do as many good repetitions as you can with the thirty pound dumbbells.

If your maximum training weight for the Dumbbell Press is less than one hundred pounds then you will not need to do as many sets.

As an example .....if you can only press the fifty pound dumbbells for five reps; then do a drop set of thirty five pound dumbbells and a last set of twenty five pound dumbbells.

Set up your dumbbells you need before you start the sets and do not cheat by resting over ten seconds at most between your drop sets.

Giant Sets

Giant Sets require performing three or more exercises ,one by one, getting only as much rest as it takes to move on to the next exercise.

This is preferably about 10 to 15 seconds ....so prepare ahead by starting your giant set workout by setting up everything you will need for your set ahead of time.

A sample of a giant set for the biceps is:

- Dumbbell Curls with forty pounds with each arm for twelve reps.

- Immediately perform reverse grip pull-up until failure.

- Immediately perform Preacher Reverse Grip Curls to failure.

Supersets

Supersets require you to perform two sets of two separate body parts, one after The other, with little or no rest in between the sets.

A sample of this for chest and biceps is:

- Dumbbell fly's immediately followed by a set of Machine Preacher Bench Curls

- Dumbbell Presses immediately followed by a set of Standing Barbell Curls

- Dumbbell pullover immediately followed by Cable Bicep Curls

Supersets keep your heart rate up while you weight train. This adds extra Many great benefits for your heart and your waist.

Supersets are great for getting a lot of work done, in as little time as possible.

Volume Training

Volume Training is the most under valued training methods for achieving great results.

I prescribe a training "cycle" using volume training for the following benefits:

- Great for developing great form and a powerful Neuro-muscular link

- Great for increasing the body's ability to pump blood into the muscles

- Increases the bodies vascularity

- Good for strengthening your tendons to prepare for heavy training stress reducing Your chances of injury

- Excellent muscle pump

- Good for developing your tolerance to lactic acid build up

- Stresses your different types of muscle fibers

There are two different repetition ranges we train between when doing Volume Training.

The first is between twenty and twenty five repetitions.

The second rep range is between twelve and fifteen repetitions.

I focus especially on my repetition speed when I do Volume Training.
I emphasize slow training whenever possible.
As per SuperSlow Principle One (covered later)

Pre-Exhaustion Training

This is a method of training where two sets are performed, one right after another. The first set is an exercise that isolates your targeted muscle..... followed by the second exercise, which is a compound movement that utilizes another entire muscle group to push the targeted muscle group in a secondary manner, further when it is impossible to do any more with the targeted muscle alone.

Here are some samples for all the different body parts:

- Flat Dumbbell fly's and Decline Chest Press

- Incline Dumbbell fly's and Incline Chest Press

- Cable fly's and Bar Dips

- Shoulder Shrugs followed by Cable Rowing

- Cable Shoulder Shrugs followed by Lat Machine Pull Downs

- Leg Extension followed by Squats

- Leg Curls with machine followed by Stiff Legged Dead Lifts

- Rear Dumbbell Laterals followed by Cable Upright Rows.

- Frontal Dumbbell Raise followed by Barbell Military Press

- Standing Donkey Raise followed by Seated Calf Raise

- Alternate Dumbbell Curls followed by Close Grip Chin Ups

The SuperSlow Protocol

Using Less Weight to Achieve Superior Results And Reduce Injury.

Gravity is what resistance or weight training is based upon.
Gravity is the force which creates the resistance required to train our body.

So it makes perfect sense to get the most out of your workout with weights that you must extract as much benefit possible through being creative with the way you work with gravity itself.

This is what I call The "SuperSlow Protocol".

The means by which you work with "SuperSlow" has to do with manipulating the speed at which we perform our repetitions during various stages of each exercise movement we do.

Each exercise ,therefore, can be broken down into two "phases" which can be applied to pretty much any and all weight training exercises.

"Phase one": is really our "pushing phase" ; the phase at which you are forcing the weight away from the ground to the half way point.

"Phase two": is the returning of your weights from the half way point and back down to the original starting point.

There are two varieties of "Phase one" applied for our purposes:

SuperSlow One (Super Slow)

Raising and lowering the weights by using a steady paced and perfectly timed fashion by counting to a specified number while you are performing the repetitions.

This is to count out 5 seconds (1 one thousand, 2 one thousand).......
while raising up the weight to finish the first "phase" of this repetition. Upon reaching the specified number of "Five" and then lowering at the same pace of 5 seconds.

SuperSlow Two (Explosive)

Accelerating or exploding against gravity for the distance traveled by the weight being lifted during the first "phase". Here the goal is to be pushing the weight as hard and as fast as possible, creating an *'acceleration'* from the starting point to the middle point (Upper point). This is the technique we
apply when using light weights ,as well as, medium resistance.

I do not find it is practical using heavy weights.
On the lowering of or returning of the weight to the starting position, we take our time and feel the muscle as we count to five
(1 one thousand, 2 one thousand).

SuperSlow down and explosive up.

Be careful not to lock your joints at the end of the acceleration movements. Near the end of the movement, as you approach the half way point, let the weight just kinda "float" up and into place.

SuperSlow Advantage Two is your new competitive edge. It has helped my clients and athletes use less weight to achieve better results with less injury.

Training Routines

Now that we have the understanding of training frequency and how it is related to performance and muscle training, we will be learning how to train to make incredible transformations to your body.

The "Four Phase" Plan is a training routine made up of several different and unique training routines that makeup an entire program.

Each training routine is a training "phase".
Each "phase" has a specific purpose and is designed to compliment the other "phases" creating a synergistic progression effect.

Or in simple terms, instead of doing the same boring program week after week and having heavier weight and sorer knees as your only means of gauging performance....The Four "phase" Plan systematically alters training stresses on the body every training "cycle".

After four different training "phases" you start at the beginning and repeat the "cycle".

We have several distinct benefits with the "Four Phase" Plan over other programs, including all of the infamous "grocery store magazine" programs.
Instead of following some set plan for twelve weeks and then simply increasing the weight and/or intensity of the exercises performed; here there is a variety of productive stresses placed upon your body that cover various redundant and specific training purposes.

I call it "Tactical Fitness" in my personal training business.
It is the workout programs that target strengthening what clients do for a living and their hobbies....While having to go the the dreaded gym anyway. The real-world client works as an insurance agent by day and plays softball by night.

This structure poses a different stimulus on your body each and every "cycle".

For several reasons this translates into incredible gains:

• Your body is put through many different forms of stimuli, more than just Increasing weights and intensity, which sooner or later cannot be continued on.

• Produces superior results for the "natural athlete" for on or off season.

• Muscular development is not just dependent on "heavy training" stimulus.

• Muscle gains are achieved with considerably less chance of injuries caused by continuous repetitive motions using very heavy weights over and over.

• All three types of muscle fibers are stimulated for maximum growth and performance.

• Plateaus occur very seldom, as the body is continually put under different training stress environments.

• Continual long term muscle gains and fat losses are much greater.

• Less gym time is required than your conventional cookie-cutter programs.

• Variety makes working out become more varied, enjoyable and not so monotonous.

• Longevity is easier to sustain by creating a mentally stimulating environment.

• Defined break periods give your body time to grow and also be transformed even more.... for continuous steady gains when you start up the next training "phase".

• Overtraining becomes very unlikely.

• Smaller muscles are focused and trained more frequently to take advantage of their ability to recuperate faster optimizing gains in strength and efficiency.

• All muscles are specialized toward your sport specific at all times.

• The "Four Phase" Plan will adapt to your specific requirements enabling Increased optimal results..... no matter what your age, training experience, or body type.

• The "Four phase" Plan is well laid-out and easy and fun to follow.

Bring it all together

Our goal in this section is to put your body through all four phases of your foundational weight and strength training.

With this knowledge we will then be able to design weight programs at a more advanced level that will focus on life, age, body type and career/health goals.

But we can not do that until we have seen your body experience the several base forms of training and their conditioning effects upon YOU.

Lets not forget what this program is 110% all about.

YOU.

11. Your Body Weight Strategy

Workouts using only your body's own weight allows you to build Agility and Strength, while combining them both together to acquire an even better state of balance and over-all physical and fitness harmony.

Being able to handle and move around your own equal body weight gives an athlete an acute sense of awareness and ruggedness when performing and executing maneuvers in a competitive setting.
This form of training allows for gains in performance far greater than the traditional "Power lifter" type trainee.......By avoiding all of the wasted tear down of the body and the associated recovery time.

Why bench press 500 pounds for a softball player, an MMA Fighter or a Cheerleader? The gains from bench pressing an amount equal to ones own "Body Weight" for a set of 15-20 reps FAR outweighs the puny gains an athlete would get from bench pressing 500 pounds one time.

Usually your competitor will be roughly the same weight as you are. Imagine the feeling of entering your next competition and KNOWING ahead of time that you can throw around your competitor as if he/she were a bag of dog food? THAT is the goal of "Body-Weight Training".
Instead of blindly bench pressing a huge amount of weight for the only goal of bench pressing 500 pounds.

This is why we will include Body-weight training in your training program.
Especially in an "On-Season" Environment.
Less recovery, Less injuries, Less breakdown, more Sport-Specific movements with more Neuro-Muscular Programming aimed at your goals.

Full body "Body-weight" workout protocol:

Three sets at 15 to 20 repetitions using YOUR body-weight....
or a percentage thereof.....while achieving 15-20 reps.

Example: If you weigh 175 pounds, then deadlift would be done with 175 pounds for a full 20 repetitions and for 3-5 sets.

Get yourself through the 3 set workout , before moving on to the 5 sets workout.

Feel free to decrease the weight, if needed, to make through all 5 sets.

If you cant do 20, then keep working this workout and doing as many reps as you can...2,10,16, whatever it may be.

Once you can effectively and correctly perform 20 reps at your body-weight.......Increase the resistance by 10%.

Example: add 15 pounds to 175 pounds in the example above....or 190.
20 reps and 5 sets.....

Repeat in future workouts , if needed.

12. Your Cardio Training

The Basics of Heart Rate Monitor Training

The goal of the vast majority of trainees is to become faster, whether the trainee is a beginner, an elite age-group (School) athlete, or a professional.

For those that have a limited amount of time, which are the majority of age-group trainees, it is essential that the time devoted towards cardio training is as productive as possible.

In order to make training time as productive as possible, it is necessary to monitor training intensity and have a means by which to gauge your training progress.

In endurance/cardio training, the means to do this include monitoring your pace, your power production, and/or your individual heart rate.
In this chapter, I will be focusing primarily on heart rate training and will devote a bit of time to pace or tempo training.

The heart rate conditioning I will be discussing will be limited to cycling and running disciplines, as these seem to be the most easily accessible to the average trainee. The road, a trail, a treadmill and/or an exercise bike are as readily available to you today, as toilet paper.

In fact , for myself, the quickest and easiest way to do long bouts of awesome low-impact cardio is to sit on my Spin Bike in front of my Big screen and watch an entire show on Netflix.
Easy 45 minutes of Steady-Pace cardio.

As for the application of the following information in this section to "Specific Sports".... Once you have the concept down with running and cycling , you will easily be able to translate the feedback to virtually ANY other activity.

The use of heart rate for Training

Using your heart rate to monitor exercise intensity is one of the easiest and least expensive methods to monitor exercise intensity. The argument against using heart rate monitors in measuring exercise intensity is that "intensity" itself is commonly referred to as a measure of energy expenditure.

Heart rate does not directly reflect your energy expenditure, in the same way as V02 (or the amount of oxygen consumed during work) or power output on the bike reflects your energy expenditure.

The two latter measurements are a direct measure of energy consumption, however you cannot measure V02 every time you train ,because it is just not practical and power output cannot be measured while you are Running.

There is a linear relationship between heart rate and V02 and your exercise intensity based on heart rate has long been considered an effective method of measuring exercise intensity and performance. We will use heart rate measurement to establish you a baseline and get a feel for where certain paces are for you specifically during certain workouts. After that we just check heart rate occasionally for comparison numbers and adjustments.

Unless, of course, you want to train with a heart rate monitor constantly?
Which is absolutely fine. These days a heart rate monitor is a $25 watch you buy at any sporting goods store.
I also have a link on the backpage to a great deal on Amazon for the one I recommend.

Heart Rate Ranges

Most trainees and trainers train within a **five heart rate Range schedule**.
These are categorized as Ranges 1 through 5.
I will be discussing how to determine your heart rate Ranges shortly, but for now I will mention they are based on your heart rate at lactate threshold (L.T.).

The Ranges and percentage of lactate threshold rate are listed below:

Range Percentage of L.T.

Range 1= anything less than 65% (Walking your dog to Brisk walking)
Range 2= 66-80% (Slow jog to medium jog)
Range 3= 81-94% (Running pace to Race pace)
Range 4= 95-101% (Competing in a race with family/friends watching)
Range 5= greater than 102% (a pack of flesh-eating Zombies is chasing you)

There are variances in the heart rate Ranges, based on lactate threshold within different coaching philosophies. In the end, the Ranges are relatively always similar regardless of the percentages based on the heart rate at threshold.

Determining Endurance Performance

Now would a good time to briefly discuss what determines endurance and/or sports performance. A great deal of research has been conducted over the past century ,investigating what makes an athlete excel in endurance performance and certain characteristics have been discovered and assigned to predict performance in endurance sports :

1.) Efficiency during performance
2.) Lactate threshold
3.) V02 max.

Efficiency is defined as an *amount of power output produced for any given amount of energy consumed*. Some exercise scientists will use the word "economy" instead of efficiency, especially when dealing with the sport of Running.
The difference is that economy is defined as *movement velocity for your given energy consumed*.

In both cases energy consumed is measured in V02 or the amount of oxygen consumed during a work bout..

Regardless of the terminology used, what is known is that the most efficient performing cyclists and economical Runners can often overcome any genetic limitations they have concerning a low V02 max. So what exactly is V02 max?

The true definition of "V02 max" is: *The greatest rate of oxygen uptake by the body.* It is dependent upon your maximum cardiac output; which is the amount of blood pumped by the heart, and the maximum arteriovenous oxygen difference, or simply put .....the amount of oxygen extracted by muscles.

When V02 max is measured in a lab, a special mask is attached to the trainee and the trainee is required to perform maximal work for a set time period. When maximal work is achieved the amount of oxygen consumed per minute is then calculated.

The infamous "V02 max" has always been considered the "Benchmark" of fitness measurements. The reason for this is because your V02 max is dependent upon the amount of blood the heart can actually pump ,or its cardiac output, and the amount of oxygen the muscles can actually extract from the blood to use for your aerobic metabolism.

Historically, it was considered that the higher your V02 max happened to be, the better the trainee performed in his or her particular sport. However, this has now been shown not to be the case. Sports physiology has evolved and numerous studies evaluated the greatest athletes performing in various sports. What was discovered was that it is not always the athlete with the greatest V02 max crossing the finish line first every time.

This should come as a relief to many trainees to learn that the actually ceiling of V02 max is genetically determined.

Once a trainee reaches a certain high level of fitness, V02 max cannot be drastically improved. What studies have shown is that the more efficient trainees are able to overcome their genetically determined lower V02 max and perform the same amount of performance with less metabolic loss.

It is the velocity at V02 max that predicts Running performance in a 3 KM time trial, for example. What has also been discovered is that some trainees are able to out-perform their competition with a higher V02 max by having a higher lactate threshold barrier.

Researchers in 2004 discovered that cardio performance of Triathletes could be precisely predicted by determining swim speed and Run speed at maximum lactate "steady-state levels".

To summarize these last two statements, is to say that..........
it is the velocity at lactate threshold that determines athletic performance.

This is *one* of the little secrets to my conditioning programs for athletes and particularly for sports trainees.
Hopefully all of the trainees reading this book just had a light go on?

This is the one secret that (up until now) no coach or trainer in sports could figure out. Why MY MMA Fighters and athletes were just "Different" during competition.

Read on......

Lactate threshold is the term used to describe the given work output performed while blood lactate increases above your "baseline" levels. Lactate is the byproduct of anaerobic metabolism by your muscles during bouts of work.

As exercise intensity starts to increase, the amount of oxygen that reaches the muscles becomes non-sufficient to allow the muscles to generate energy using oxygen, or aerobic metabolism. At this point the muscles are required to produce energy via anaerobic, or without oxygen, means.

As the intensity of your workout increases, the amount of lactate produced increases, and due to changes in the flow of blood, the removal of lactate decreases.

A certain point is reached in which lactate production increases beyond a state of lactate removal and the blood lactate concentration increases quite considerably.

This is your "lactate threshold" point.

A person's lactate threshold is the approximate intensity of exercise that can be maintained steadily for one hour.

I will clarify the previous statement by saying that there is a variation in how long a trainee can perform at their individual lactate threshold and there are also many factors that must be considered when stating how long a trainee can continue performing at lactate threshold intensity levels.

Regardless of this fact, the higher a trainee's lactate threshold is in relation to his V02 max, the higher the intensity of exercise that can be maintained.

Now if we bring heart rate specifics of performance together we can discuss how these specifics can be interrelated.

Visualize the V02 max as the size of the engine in an automobile.
The higher the V02 max, equals the bigger the engine and the larger the potential of power to be output.

Now picture the lactate threshold as the "red line" limitations of the RPM gauge. If the engine produces maximal power output at 6,000 RPM (or for the trainee at 170 beats per minute of heart rate), but redlines at 4,000 RPM (or 140 beats per minute heart rate), the high V02 max is not the true limitations on your performance.

The trainee cannot even come close to V02 max and its intensities.
For the most part, a usable lactate threshold of 80% of V02 max is considered quite good.

Where does efficiency come into play?

In the human body, efficiency is developed in part by the economy of movement and partially by the genetic make-up of the human body.

Economy in Running is related to qualities such as a high stride rate and using mid-foot or forefoot Running.

If two Runners have identical V02 max and lactate threshold at 78% of V02 max ; one Runner could Run at a 5 minute per mile pace and the other Runner at a 7 minute per mile pace solely due to a difference in each of their "Running economy" or "Efficiency of performance".

Efficiency in cycling refers to a smooth pedal stroke, while pedaling in perfect circles, ankling, and exact cadence for a given power output.

In Swimming, efficiency is the most critical of the performance sports and deals with a smooth and streamlined series of strokes.

Adapting this information to your desired need or want for physical qualities of "efficiency" is really quite easy; as you can see.

Training within Determined "Ranges"

Range 1 is used primarily for recovery, building resistance to fatigue during long training sessions and for working on training your overall efficiency.

Range 2 is primarily used for your endurance training.
The intensity of this Range is sufficient to produce cardiovascular improvement with conditioning and time, yet not intensive enough to severely break down any one part of the body during training.

Range 3 is a higher intensity used for a more intensive form endurance training. This is the Range commonly used for tempo training workouts. This level of intensity stimulates more cardiovascular benefits to the athlete than Range 2, however the volume of Range 3 training needs to be limited (especially Running) due to the stresses imposed on the body with this intensity of this training.

This is why here and beyond....We focus a lot of attention on swimming and spin-bike.

Range 4 is primarily used for "lactate threshold conditioning" work.
This level is just below or at a trainee's lactate threshold baseline.
This is quite serious training and is both physically and psychologically stressing.

It is generally used only once per week during structured training in the "off-season/no-competition" phases of training.

This range of training should be limited due to the high risk of injury and long-term breakdown of the joints and ligaments.

Range 5 is used to train a trainee's V02 max and should be used very rarely, especially while Running, due to the extreme stresses on the body.

Once an trainee has achieved a high level of cardiovascular fitness, V02 max intervals should be used very sparingly.

As I have already mentioned, V02 max is genetically determined and once the ceiling of V02 max is reached, it cannot then be increased drastically.

Training time should be spent elsewhere. The exception, is cycling in which we can increase power at V02 max.

A final statement regarding these training ranges.......
 as you progress from Range 1 and through the ranges to Range 5, the percentage of fat supplying body its fuel to burn ***decreases*** and the percentage of carbohydrates supplying fuel to the working muscles **increases**.

The point?

Range 2 to 3 are generally your "Burning Fat" range.

Range 3 to 4 are your range for conditioning.

Range 5 is then your "Competition or Simulation" range.

Determining your heart rate Ranges

The next topic I will discuss is how to determine your heart rate Ranges for your training. The most valid method of determining heart rate training range is a lactate threshold test on the treadmill or cycle computer.

Lactate threshold testing involves increasing the workload in stages and obtaining blood samples at the end of each of these stages.

There are numerous field tests which can be done to estimate lactate threshold for cycling and/or Running. If a laboratory lactate threshold test cant be performed (9 times out of 10 this is the case), the best method of determining lactate threshold heart rate is via a 30 minute time trial on the bike followed by a 30 minute Run at threshold to race pace (4.5 to 5).

To determine lactate threshold heart rate, measure the average heart rate for the entire event. It is best that these are as close to actual race paces in order to maximize accurate results.

Once your lactate threshold heart rate has been determined, training can be focused around that lactate threshold. When the lactate threshold test has been performed , the maximum effort is usually reached in order to evaluate maximum heart rate. Maximum heart rate does correspond with V02 max heart rate, however V02 max cannot be determined without specialized metabolic equipment.

Either way, you can take a look at the lactate threshold heart rate and V02 max heart rate and determine your percentage within practical use.

If lactate threshold heart rate is above 70%-80% of V02 max, but your Run velocity is slow and we are dealing with a highly trained athlete, time and practice should be spent working on run economy.

If the trainee is young in terms of training age, training could be focused on VO2 max and Running economy.

If the lactate threshold heart rate is below 70% of VO2 max heart rate, then training should be focused on lactate threshold

The training objectives should also be considered based on the training season (on/off or competition, etc.) and training age of the trainee.

Monitoring your training stress

Another benefit of training using heart rate is the benefit of effective monitoring of your training stress/load.
Effective training protocols take into account your volume, frequencies and the intensity of the particular training.

Training without a heart rate monitor allows you to easily measure volume and frequency with a calendar and watch, but training intensity will be difficult to monitor without a heart rate monitor.

Your heart rate is a measure of exercise intensity. By measuring heart rate and duration of the work session, training values can be calculated and used as an integrative measure of exercise load during training and competition.

Heart rate Training does have its Shortcomings

We will now look at some drawbacks to training by using your heart rate.
The first issue is that the heart rate is not always your most valid indicator of exercise intensity.

For example, on a training Run performed at an 8-minute per mile pace, a trainee's heart rate may be 140bpm on one given day. On another day, an 8-minute per mile pace may yield a heart rate of 150bpm.

This can be a good measure of training intensity, or it can be quite misleading. If a person is sick, dehydrated, injured, or etc.... It would be very likely in the trainee's best interest to modify this workout or call it a day and focus on his/her recovery.

The training heart rate is a valid measure of body-stress and should be used to monitor exercise intensity.
Alternatively, it can also be an invalid measure of stress.

For example, if the trainee is racing today and the excitement of the race is "artificially" driving up his heart rate due to hormone release, the heart rate should be ignored and other measures of monitoring the intensity should be implemented.
This would be construed as a rating of perceived exertion or pace.

Finally, another topic when it comes to monitoring heart rate in endurance training is the topic of "Cardiac Drift".

The definition of **cardiac drift** would be an increase in heart rate over time at the same exact intensity. I can confidently state that every trainee reading this article has experienced some form of cardiac drift.

A common example would be an hour (or even longer) training Run.
At the start of the Run you are happily running 9-minute miles with a heart rate of 155bpm.

You decide you will maintain the run pace at 9 minutes per mile, but at about mile 6 you begin to notice your heart rate is 160bpm. Has your intensity increased?
Based upon pace, no....... but in terms of physiology, YES.

Historically, the underlying reason for cardiac drift had been considered to be from dehydration.

However, in recent research it has been shown that cardiac drift cannot be prevented by sufficient hydration alone.

Obviously, there are training sessions in which a certain pace or power intensity is desired with no regard to your heart rate, however those training sessions have certain and different specific goals. Other factors that can affect heart rate are caffeine or drugs, altitude, and/or bodily hormones.

Depending on your particular circumstances, training by heart rate when under the influences of the above, might or might not require adjustment of training Ranges or using other methods of monitoring your training intensity.

Training by using Pace

Training by pace versus heart rate. Training Ranges based on your pace can be calculated based on recent race results or laboratory lactate threshold tests and various different field tests.

At the initial start of a training session, heart rate and running pace correlate very closely; however, as mentioned before, as the training session continues cardiac drift will occur and maintaining the same running pace will yield a higher heart rate.

A major 2005 study revealed that heart rate should be monitored, as it is a relatively accurate indicator of metabolic intensity. However, there is considerable debate regarding this topic. In cycling, just as advanced research has supported that "even pacing" for optimum time trial performance is best.

I would personally suggest caution when training and competing based purely on pace alone. I suggest using several methods for monitoring your training and competition intensity.

When coaching my athletes, I generally prescribe training/racing by Run pace for those with a very large base of training miles and done for only specific workouts to mimic their race pace. This is only done when the training environment is known.

I will also mention another very important benefit of training by pace. When training by pace, the trainee is required to achieve some certain desired pace, thus the training economy is being reinforced.

A common mistake I see trainees make when training by heart rate alone, is the achieving a desired heart rate level due to inefficiency or sloppiness.

This is easily seen when your pace at two different training Ranges are identical ,or at the very least, very similar. Training by pace does circumvent this potential training problem.

In the last few years a growing number of athletes have shifted to using power to monitor and pace their training sessions and races. Training by power has quite a few benefits.

However, in my professional opinion, training by power alone should not be done exclusively and it is most effective when incorporating heart rate based training and monitoring along with.

Benefits of Power-Based Training

There are many benefits of training using power as your guide.
One of the most practical reasons for training by using power is that you can dial-in your short intervals and immediately ensure you are training at the proper training Ranges.

An example of this is the use of intervals in " Range 5 ", where we are training at improving V02max/Peak Power Output.
If a trainee is training by heart rate methods alone, he may under-estimate or over-estimate the intensity of this short interval workout due to the fact that heart rate does not instantaneously increase when power is also increased.
This is known as **heart rate lag**.

Oftentimes one is nearly complete with the interval before heart rate reaches a steady state ,which can take up to 3+ minutes, and the interval is completed long before the trainee realizes he or she has over or under exerted the interval.

This is also particularly obvious while training for sprint or neuromuscular power and when training by heart rate is impossible due to the shortness of the intervals.

Also, power-based training can be used to calculate training stresses and ensure training is progressive in nature, adding adequate stress at appropriate times and more importantly insuring adequate recovery.

One of the other benefits of power-based training is that it is very easy to track your fitness-level improvements. You can compare the average power during the interval and compare the power to your average heart rate and vice-versa.

With the proper training, power output will be increased at a given heart rate. This is quite evident with cycling performance, as tracking speed at a given heart rate is highly variable due to temperature, course variations, wind, terrain, and etc..

On a another note, training by power also allows you to record your efforts for future use. For example, you may race on a particular course one day and note the average power output for that course.

At a later date you race the exact same course and have a different finish time. Was your race better or worse?

By evaluating your power data, you can decide how you progressed or weakened. Heart rate data alone would not tell us this. With our power data we can evaluate our strengths and weaknesses more precisely.

Explosive Power Training and its Benefit to a trainee

When there is recorded data that you can compare your power output for a given length of time (example: 5 second, 5 minute, 20 minute, etc.) to the average power output in a given category of cyclists (example: Cat 1 or 2, Cat 3, etc.) It will become more evident that sprinting ability is actually quite important for trainees.

A trainee will likely never sprint in their specific sport; however, the concept of your power reserve is very important for a trainee, as a power reserve has been shown to be a more useful predictor of performance than is the V02max in time trial performance.

One of the difficulties I frequently encounter with trainees is the ability to "hammer" the intensity up. Power-based training allows one to track the progression of peak power for different time intervals.

An quick analogy of how increasing your power reserve can help your time trial performance may help.

Two trainees are performing the squat exercise with weights.
One trainee has a one-repetition maximum of 450 pounds while the other trainee has a one-repetition maximum of 250 pounds.

While both trainees can squat 250 pounds 20 repetitions; one can speculate that squatting 225 pounds 20 repetitions will be more stressful for that trainee with the one repetition maximum of 250 pounds compared to the trainee that has a one-repetition maximum of 450 pounds.

This can be generalized to ALL sports performance.

If two trainees have virtually identical heart rate threshold power outputs of 315 Watts, yet one trainee has a peak power output of 500 Watts and the other trainee has a peak power output of 600 Watts, one can speculate the trainee with the greater peak power output will be less "stressed" while performing at that heart rate threshold .....assuming using the same training volume and/or practice.

The generalized training practice for coaching and training trainees has been to focus on the volume portion and to maintain training intensity *below* heart rate threshold.

However, research and experience show us that this may not be the optimal training practice and that by adding explosive strength training and sprinting to the training practice , you can yield better endurance performance.
This due perhaps via increased efficiency and increased heart rate threshold power, and I would also dare to speculate that this is also due to improved power reserve.

Recent research has discovered that replacing a portion of endurance training with explosive style resistance training, while at the same time maintaining overall training volume, can lead to an improved time trial performances.

Benefits of Training by using your heart rate

The benefit of heart rate training includes the ability to factor in what is taking place in the trainee's entire body.

Example: Let's say a trainee normally relies on the power method for pacing training intervals and the trainee based the power intervals from a testing of his performance on an ideal day where the temperature was 75-degrees and humidity was 30% and the trainee felt fantastic.

However on a different training day it is 98 degrees with 80% humidity. It will be very difficult for the trainee to be able to maintain the same performance on this hotter and more humid day compared to the ideal conditions day.

Heart rate monitoring will help you take into account the training performance for the different training days based on the trainee's condition and the environmental conditions.

Benefits of R.P.E. training (AKA: Rating of perceived Exertion)

R.P.E. has been used since before the advent of using heart rate monitors and power meters to gauge progress. Training by R.P.E. could be viewed as less specific as training by using heart rate and power measures.

R.P.E. could be used under certain situations. As an example, during the early stages of a Triathlon race.... heart rate may not feel in-line with the effort due to the "Race day" excitement experienced by the trainee.

In this instance, R.P.E. may be a very valid method of pacing.
R.P.E. is a useful alternative when conditions are present that will affect pace and overall performance
(i.e. hills, wind, environment induced extremes, etc).

Benefits of Training using a Combination of heart rate, Power, and R.P.E.

My training method combines power-based training, heart rate training, and the use of rating of perceived exertion. There are many trainers out there that preach some form of power-based training as the perfect form of training, however this goes against exercise physiology principles on many different levels. Power-based training is truly valuable when it is combined with heart rate ,as well as, R.P.E. training.

When training short intervals power-based training ensures the trainee is achieving the proper Ranges of training. Also, progress can be assessed by evaluating duration a trainee is maintaining a given power output, for example, perform repeat sessions at various power output to determine critical power and evaluate fitness improvement.

Also, for comparing power output to heart rate. With training, this leads to an overall increased power output at a given heart rate.

A valid training program should not be based on training by power or heart rate alone, but should take into account power, heart rate, and perceived exertion. It is acknowledged that not every trainee has a power type device or computer.

Cyclists have been training for over a century without power-training devices. What is more important is that you take full advantage of your training devices, whether it is a power meter or heart rate monitor. Simply looking down at a power meter or heart monitor will not automatically lead to any fitness improvement.

Tempo Cardio Vs. Steady-State Cardio

Whether for competition or just for your personal enrichment; endurance, effort and speed are the most important components of your "Cardio training".

When you're training a long or unknown distance or time, we use the tempo cardio technique. It allows you to maintain a relatively even and stable pace and heart rate throughout the work bout, regardless of the distance or time.

Shorter distance or times -- like a 5k -- benefit more from steady-state Running, however, a slow-and-steady pace can really work for any type of distance.

Tempo Training

According to "Running Times," the original definition of a tempo Run originated from Jack Daniels' Running Formula (also the premise for most of my cardio training practices).

According to the Daniels formula, tempo Running equals

"20 minutes of steady Running at heart rate threshold pace."

Your heart rate-threshold pace should be conversationally/comfortably hard -- a pace you could maintain for about one hour or so.

We sometimes refer to as "Conversational pace", or a pace where a a training partner and yourself could keep up a talk while working out.

During training, the body breaks down carbohydrates for use as energy. As these carbohydrates are metabolized by the body, lactate is produced as a byproduct. Up to a certain point, the body can clear-out the lactate as quickly as it is produced.

Tempo training involves performing at an effort level *just below* the point where the body can no longer keep up with the lactate production. At this work level, lactate does not accumulate -- and the body can withstand a longer workout.

This is why one of the first things I like to do is have a young trainee begin training to compete in the local "5K races" in their local communities. 5K ONLY and no further! You can see why as we read further.

Tempo Pace

Each trainee's tempo pace varies according to his or her level of cardio.
The proper "Tempo Running" pace is roughly 25 to 30 seconds per mile *slower* than your current 5k racing pace.

For more advanced Runners, a tempo running pace would be somewhere around a 10 mile pace.

Whether "Running" or performing some other workout...... If you're using a heart rate monitor, tempo training should keep your heart rate relatively consistent at 90 percent of your maximum heart rate.

Steady-State Training

Steady-state is quite similar to tempo training. However, Steady-state training also takes the lactate threshold into consideration. With steady-state training, your effort level should be drastically lower than the point where the body can no longer keep up with lactate production.

While steady-state training, your fatigue should occur from the **duration** of the workout and not from your speed, as it is with Tempo training.

Steady-State Pace

A steady-state training pace is somewhere between a level where the pace can be held for *25* to *75* minutes.

A steady-state workout should maintain a relatively consistent heart rate between 80 and 85 percent of your maximum heart rate on your heart rate monitor.

One of my famous trademark techniques for this one is having my clients use the swimming Pool.
No matter what level of swimmer you are.

In fact, the worse your swimming skills are, the better the workout actually is.
Yes I realize the defies the rules of efficiency, however in the pool their is little risk of injury to joints or ligaments.
Even if you need the floaties or kickboard.
Even if you back stroke and doggy paddle.

20+ minutes of swimming is the BEST use of your "Steady State" Cardio training time per week. So much so that I'd bet a 5K PR Medal around your neck on it.

Cardio Machine Training

Not good weather out side to train?
Dont like Walking or Running outdoors? To much traffic?
No excuses needed.

Cardio Machine training doesn't have to be mind-numbing and /or boring.
A repertoire of creative workouts can allow you to both have fun and drastically increase your fitness heart rate and performance levels.

I use the term "Machine" for simplicity, because all of this info applies to a Spin bike, Elliptical or other cardio machine.

Land running vs. Cardio Machine

In treadmill and machine training you don't have to overcome resistance from wind, because you stay in the same spot.

As a result, you need to set a treadmill to 1 percent incline to approximate the 7 percent energy cost you usually use to overcome air resistance.

Second, in machine training, the ground "moves out" from underneath you instead of you pushing against the ground to propel yourself over the ground. As a result, your biomechanics are slightly off or different.

Since there are no curves or bumps or curves in the surface ,your footplant or ground connection is exactly the same nearly every stride or movement. Take care when starting treadmill and machine workouts to let your body adjust to the different demands.

You need to gradually introduce machine to your routine, and it's a good idea to do some preparatory easy workouts before you do machine training.

"Cruise Intervals" or Speed Play

A Fartlek (Swedish term for "speed play") is a High Intensity Cardio workout followed by a timed bout of Lower Intensity Cardio work, for example sprinting and jogging off and on during a training Run.

A normal workout is a 20-60 minute constant training session.

Using Fartlek ,instead of keeping the same pace and heart rate throughout the entire workout , you take the intensity "UP and DOWN" (for example sprint, then jog, then sprint again) whenever you feel like it.

You can customize a fartlek workout to however you feel. If you feel sluggish today, limit the number of sprints you actually do, and take a little more time to recover.

If you arent feeling great, UP the intensity hard for a set time or distance and back DOWN and don't sprint again until you feel totally recovered.

Speed Play can be performed while Swimming, Running, Treadmill, Biking, walking, or anywhere or in any sport where movement is performed. Remember this information as we proceed into "Sport Specific" drills and workouts much later on in our programs.

One good way to perform this type of workout is to pick out objects ahead of you during a Run or a bike, like a telephone pole, and go 'level 4' from that pole to the next and then back to 'level 2'.
Or a point of time ahead on the clock, so as to be "Racing the clock".
One reason that fartleks are so popular is that it is so flexible of a workout.

Before starting a fartlek, make sure that you warm up at least 10-15 minutes to ensure that your muscles are loosened-up enough to handle the accelerations and decelerations.

Also, a cool down 10-15 minutes after the workout.
The fartlek can be a quite difficult workout, and if you don't warm up and cool down properly, you could have some very sore muscles the next day.

Starting to do fartleks can be tough on your body if it isn't ready for the faster paces used during the workout.

After the workout, it is also very important to refuel your body by drinking water and eating protein-rich foods to get the most benefits and to help your muscle recovery.

Although fartlek's popularity is due in part to its flexibility of use, many trainers like to make the workout more structured and give it more of a "track interval-type" feel.

A structured fartlek workout might be:

10 minute warm up, 2 minutes hard, 2 minutes easy, 3 minutes hard, 3 minutes easy, 4 minutes hard, 4 minutes easy, 4 minutes hard, 3 minutes easy, 3 minutes hard, 2 minutes easy, 2 minutes hard, 15 minutes cool down.

This workout would be labeled by calling it a: 2, 3, 4, 3, 2.

Brining it all together

Our overall goal with cardio right now is to explore what options are not only available to you, but what you can actually DO on a regular basis......THEN from that we are looking for what actually works for you and what the prescribed times and doses are going to be.

Some people can look like a soap opera star with only two 20 minute workouts in the pool per week......But fall to pieces when they try to run heavy miles and lift heavy weights. Some people may perform like a champion with a steady regime of weight training and a lot of machine cardio.....But swimming and interval training not so much.

It all depends on the individual.

That is the goal of this entire program. YOU!

I can not stress this point enough.

So experiment with cardio.
You may find that an hour a week is all you ever need....if you go to the pool.

13. Constructing your "Fitness Plan"

By now you know that your strategic fitness program, you will need to cover five major areas of focus

1.) Flexibility
2.) Endurance
3.) Strength
4.) Power
5.) Anaerobic

Regardless of your current age or physical/fitness condition, your overall fitness program needs to address and plan for each of these areas.

Of course I am just like you....... I definitely enjoy some areas much more than others. But all areas need to be addressed.

Each of these areas need not be addressed daily.
In fact most of your major muscle groups require at least 48 hours of recovery when exercised at a high intensity. And 48 hours is for Pros and advanced.

"Overtraining" causes injury. In fact......Most gym-ending , as well as, career-ending injuries these days are a result of "over use Issues" in my opinion.
As I have stated repeatedly. Listen to and learn your body.
What exercises for what goal. What foods for this effect on the body......or prevent an effect upon my body. Learn when to "go hard" or "go soft" or not go at all (in a good way).

The major components will , however, need to be worked at least two times a week.
Endurance, Flexibility and Anaerobic will require a little more frequent work.

To get the full benefits of the HGH release....
Muscle burn , oxygen debt, elevated body temperature and adrenal response needs / must occur on as many days per week as possible.
Notice I didnt say " You must nearly kill yourself everyday"?
Do NOT overtrain.

Specific workouts have been laid out in the chapters of this manual and examples given on the website. In the "Action Phase" of this program (Next)........I have laid out custom programs designed specifically for the sport or activity performed. The drills, exercises, stretches, diets and etc primarily only vary by age and fitness level. If some one with a lower fitness level is unable to perform a program prescribed exercise do to handicap, injury or etc.....He/She would just simply replace that exercise with another one from the libraries of other choices. The choice corresponding as closely as possible to the exercise being replaced , yet still functional without pain or injury.

You will also be given a choice to have me personally review you and your goals and situation. This is where I design your program for you from a coaches perspective....to get you started on your lifelong fitness journey.

Interested in a Custom Program?

Tracking Your Progress With The Program Logs

Your Strategic Fitness Program will also be your training logs for tracking your progress. Logs are provided for Diet/Nutrition, Sleep and of course....
your workouts in the 5 components listed above.

By charting and writing down your fitness progress levels in your logs every day, you will be able to track your successes and fails in all of aspects of your eventual winning physical level.

The keys to program success are:
1.) Plan your work
2.) Work your plan
3.) Record your results

Our Programs are designed to attack one workout at a time and doing it all one week at a time.
At the beginning of the week, plan your training schedule for that entire week. And after each workout, review and update your logs....So you can keep your goals and progress within sight.

Shock Training & Muscle memory

Personal Trainers, Bobybuilders and athletes all experienced in resistance training all understand how "muscle memory" works. They have all learned the value of "shocking" their muscles during workouts to pull themselves out of any plateaus they may hit.

Decades of scientific and gym research shows that a 12-week Program and then a switch to another form of training, or new exercises or different intensities or etc......For another 12-weeks......Is what works best to maximize progress from a trainee.
Basically, every season we need to change-up the program in some way shape or form. Of course we focus these changes on our specific purpose and goals, but change the program enough to break-up in monotony the body has put itself into.

DIET and NUTRITION

Please go to my Amazon Store to purchase all of your supplements and supplies. I have found the best deals on the same stuff you'll by at the store....Only cheaper and delivered to your front door. Using the #1 and most trusted retailer on the planet.

Supplies

In Closing

If you encounter any Issues or have any questions or want a processional coach with thousands of past clients and decades of experience to review and design your program for you.........

Just purchase a Training Session!

14. **SECTION II (The Action Plan)**

15. Your Year Long Nutritional Plan

DIET PLAN: MONTH 1 , 2 AND 3

	Monday	Tuesday	Wednes	Thursda	Friday	Saturday
Meal 1	Meal #1 Meat / Carb -Balanced-	Meal #1 Meat / Carb -Balanced-	Meal #1 Meat / Carb -Balanced-	Meal #1 Meat / Carb -Balanced-	Meal #1 Meat / Carb -Balanced-	Meal #1 Meat / Carb -Balanced-
Meal 2	Meal #2	Meal #2	Meal #2	Meal #2	Meal #2	Meal #2
Meal 3	Meal #3 Veggie Heavy	Meal #3 Veggie Heavy	Meal #3 Veggie Heavy	Meal #3 Veggie Heavy	Meal #3 Veggie Heavy	Meal #3 Veggie Heavy
Meal 4	SNACK	SNACK	SNACK	SNACK	SNACK	SNACK
Meal 5	Shake	Shake	Shake	Shake	Shake	Shake
Meal 6	Shake	Shake	Shake	Shake	Shake	Shake
Meal 7	Shake	Shake	Shake	Shake	Shake	Shake
Meal 8	Low-Carb Shake	Low-Carb Shake	Low-Carb Shake	Low-Carb Shake	Low-Carb Shake	Low-Carb Shake

Sunday is "OPEN". Eat wisely, but enjoy the day
Sunday is "FAST". Get in your cardio and do not eat until 5PM

DIET PLAN: MONTH 4, 5 AND 6

	Monday	Tuesday	Wednes	Thursda	Friday	Saturday
Meal 1	Shake	Shake	Shake	Shake	Shake	Shake
Meal 2	Shake	Shake	Shake	Shake	Shake	Shake
Meal 3	Shake	Shake	Shake	Shake	Shake	Shake
Meal 4	Shake	Shake	Shake	Shake	Shake	Shake
Meal 5	Shake	Shake	Shake	Shake	Shake	Shake
Meal 6	Shake	Shake	Shake	Shake	Shake	Shake
Meal 7	Meal #1 Meat / Carb -Balanced-	Meal #1 Meat / Carb -Balanced-	Meal #1 Meat / Carb -Balanced-	Meal #1 Meat / Carb -Balanced-	Meal #1 Meat / Carb -Balanced-	Meal #1 Meat / Carb -Balanced-
Meal 8	Meal #3 Veggie Heavy	Meal #3 Veggie Heavy	Meal #3 Veggie Heavy	Meal #3 Veggie Heavy	Meal #3 Veggie Heavy	Meal #3 Veggie Heavy

Sunday is "OPEN". Eat wisely, but enjoy the day
Sunday is "FAST". Get in your cardio and do not eat until 5PM

DIET PLAN: MONTH 7 , 8 AND 9

	Monday	Tuesday	Wednes	Thursda	Friday	Saturday
Meal 1	Meal #1 Meat / Carb -Balanced-	Meal #1 Meat / Carb -Balanced-	Meal #1 Meat / Carb -Balanced-	Meal #1 Meat / Carb -Balanced-	Meal #1 Meat / Carb -Balanced-	Meal #1 Meat / Carb -Balanced-
Meal 2	Meal #2	Meal #2	Meal #2	Meal #2	Meal #2	Meal #2
Meal 3	SNACK	SNACK	SNACK	SNACK	SNACK	SNACK
Meal 4	Meal #3 Veggie Heavy	Meal #3 Veggie Heavy	Meal #3 Veggie Heavy	Meal #3 Veggie Heavy	Meal #3 Veggie Heavy	Meal #3 Veggie Heavy
Meal 5	Shake	Shake	Shake	Shake	Shake	Shake
Meal 6	Shake	Shake	Shake	Shake	Shake	Shake
Meal 7	Shake	Shake	Shake	Shake	Shake	Shake
Meal 8	Low-Carb Shake	Low-Carb Shake	Low-Carb Shake	Low-Carb Shake	Low-Carb Shake	Low-Carb Shake

Sunday is "OPEN". Eat wisely, but enjoy the day
Sunday is "FAST". Get in your cardio and do not eat until 5PM

DIET PLAN: MONTH 10, 11 AND 12

	Monday	Tuesday	Wednes	Thursda	Friday	Saturday
Meal 1	Shake	Shake	Shake	Shake	Shake	Shake
Meal 2	Meal #1 Meat / Carb -Balanced-	Meal #1 Meat / Carb -Balanced-	Meal #1 Meat / Carb -Balanced-	Meal #1 Meat / Carb -Balanced-	Meal #1 Meat / Carb -Balanced-	Meal #1 Meat / Carb -Balanced-
Meal 3	Shake	Shake	Shake	Shake	Shake	Shake
Meal 4	Meal #2	Meal #2	Meal #2	Meal #2	Meal #2	Meal #2
Meal 5	Shake	Shake	Shake	Shake	Shake	Shake
Meal 6	SNACK	SNACK	SNACK	SNACK	SNACK	SNACK
Meal 7	Shake	Shake	Shake	Shake	Shake	Shake
Meal 8	Meal #3 Veggie Heavy	Meal #3 Veggie Heavy	Meal #3 Veggie Heavy	Meal #3 Veggie Heavy	Meal #3 Veggie Heavy	Meal #3 Veggie Heavy

Sunday is "OPEN". Eat wisely, but enjoy the day
Sunday is "FAST". Get in your cardio and do not eat until 5PM

16. Your Year Long Cardio Plan

Cardio Plan: Month 1 , 2 and 3

	3 Mile -or- 30 Minutes	4 Mile -or- 40 Minutes	5 Mile -or- 50 Minutes	NOTES:
Week 1	(12:38)			
Week 2				
Week 3				
Week 4				
Week 5				
Week 6				
Week 7				
Week 8				
Week 9				
Week 10				
Time Trial				

Level 2 or "Steady State" intensity. A pace you can maintain for a 45 minutes to an hour. These are you Long Slow Distance workouts.

AT THE END OF THIS CYCLE **be sure to do a "Time Trial" in each Run or "Distance traveled" on equipment.**

Cardio Plan: Month 4, 5 and 6

	2 Mile	3 Mile	4 Mile	1 Mile
Week 1	(12:38)			
Week 2				
Week 3				
Week 4				Trial
Week 5				
Week 6				
Week 7				
Week 8				Trial
Week 9				
Week 10				
Time Trial				

Level 3-4 of intensity. If your BEST 1 mile time is 8 minutes....Your average for these runs would be about 9. Best 1 mile is 10 minutes....Pace would be 11-ish. This is NOT race pace. Stay under the "puke zone".

AT THE END OF THIS CYCLE be sure to do a "Time Trial" in each Run or "Distance traveled" on equipment.

Cardio Plan: Month 7 , 8 and 9

	3 miles or 30 minutes	2 miles or 20 minutes	4 miles or 40 minutes	
Week 1	(12:38)			
Week 2				
Week 3				
Week 4				
Week 5				
Week 6				
Week 7				
Week 8				
Week 9				
Week 10				
Time Trial				

'Speed Play' at will, however the goal of these workouts IS to get 4-8 "100 yard Sprints" into the run times/distances.

AT THE END OF THIS CYCLE **be sure to do a "Time Trial" in each Run or "Distance traveled" on equipment.**

TREADMILL or RUN Cardio Plan: Alternate and Bad Weather

	15 minutes or 1.5 miles	20 minutes or 2 miles	30 minutes or 3 miles	10 min EZ :30 Sprint X 3
Week 1	(12:38)			
Week 2				
Week 3				
Week 4				
Week 5				
Week 6				
Week 7				
Week 8				
Week 9				
Week 10				
Time Trial				

Alternate between jogging, Sprinting and walking. Once the distance can be covered in "10 minutes per mile". Begin jogging the distances and throwing in bouts of sprinting. Also see the section on "Optional Workouts" if/when you have progressed passed this cardio repertoire.

AT THE END OF THIS CYCLE be sure to do a "Time Trial" in each Run or "Distance traveled" on equipment.

Cardio Plan: TreadMill alternative

	20 Minutes at level 2-3	20 minutes alternating sprints	30 Minutes at level 2-3	30 minutes alternating sprints
Week 1	(12:38)			
Week 2				
Week 3				
Week 4				
Week 5				
Week 6				
Week 7				
Week 8				
Week 9				
Week 10				
Time Trial	1 MILE			

Use the SPEED feature on the treadmill to control your difficulty, otherwise remain at a comfort yet stressed pace that is only a bit difficult for you.

The real "Killer portion" should be the SPRINTS. Breathe/Stress level= 3-4.

4 minutes jog and 1 minute Sprint is a good formula to start with.

AT THE END OF THIS CYCLE be sure to do a "Time Trial" in each Run or "Distance traveled" on equipment.

17. Your Year Long Strength Plan

Month 1 , 2 and 3

Exercise	Set 1	Set 2	Set 3		
Barbell Chest Press					
Bent-Over Barbell Row					
Barbell Narrow Grip Bicep Curl					
Overhead Barbell Press					
Bench Dips using Weight Plate on lap for weight					
Windshield Wipers followed immediately by Abdominal Atomix					
Ass-To-Grass Low Squat (Literally as low as you go)					

H.I.T. Protocol : Near your maximum 1 repetition maximum
1 to 3 repetitions per set

Month 4, 5 and 6

Exercise	Set 1	Set 2	Set 3		
DumbBell Incline Fly					
Wide Lat Pull-Downs					
DumbBell Seated Curl					
DumbBell Shoulder lateral raises. (Straight arms) I use 10's!					
Dips					
Leg Extension immediately followed by Leg Curls					
Lying Toe Touches immediately followed by Cross Crunches					

Volume Protocol: 60% of the weight from your 1 repetition maximum
15-20 repetitions per set

Month 7, 8 and 9

Exercise	Set 1	Set 2	Set 3		DROP by 50%
DumbBell Chest Press					To FAIL
BarBell Dead Lift					
Wide grip BarBell Curl					
DumbBell Military Press					
Cable Tricep Pushdowns					
Leg Press					
Abdominal Machine					

Drop Set Protocol: Exactly like your H.I.T. workout was BUT......
on your LAST set (Set 3) put your drop set in with 60% of 1 repetition max (Set 1 and 2) for 15 to 20 repetitions.

Month 10, 11 and 12

Exercise	Set 1	Set 2	Set 3		SS
DumbBell Incline Press					**5 up 5 down**
Strict Hyper-Extension with Light DumbBell					**5 up 5 down**
Preacher bench Curls with curl bar					**5 up 5 down**
BarBell Behind the Neck Military Press					**5 up 5 down**
Dumbbell Behind-the-neck Overhead Tricep Press (One D/B)					**5 up 5 down**
Incline Sit-up Board: Arms extended above head Sit-Ups					**5 up 5 down**
Leg Curls Followed immediately by Leg Extensions					**5 up 5 down**

Super Slow Protocol: All repetitions are done with a FIVE count down and a FIVE count back up.

18. Your Year Long Conditioning and Drills Plan

Workout " A "

DRILL	Set 1	Set 2	Set 3		
<u>Alternating Side Kicks (Left lead and Right)</u> In fight position throw waist level side kick. Pull back and repeat. 50 then switch lead leg.					
<u>Alternating In-Place Lunges</u> with Jab + Cross (1-2) at the top position Repeat for 1 minute.					
<u>Plank while alternating knees forward</u> while in plank position, bring knees forward and to the side. Alternate legs. 1 Minute.					
<u>In-Place alternating Lunges</u> Hands in fight position, put right leg forward and drop into lunge. Hold at bottom. 1-2 punch. Up and switch. Repeat for 1 minute.					
<u>Plank while alternating donkey kicks</u> while in plank position , pull in foot as far as possible & then kick out as far and high as possible. 1 Minute.					

Workout " B "

DRILL	Set 1	Set 2	Set 3		
Standing Bicycle Standing str8 as possible, touch right elbow to left knee at about the half way point on your body. Repeat for 1 minute.					
Squat with alternating Sidekick regular in place squat. At top position perform right side kick. Repeat squat and kick with left. and so forth. 1 Minute					
In-Place jumping Lead Changes in fight position throw a 1-2 punch , then using calves & quads, jump while switching your forward foot from right to left. Repeat for 1 minute.					
Plank while alternating donkey kicks while in plank position , pull in foot as far as possible & then kick out as far and high as possible. 1 Minute.					
Punch Kick Burpee Combos Fight position, punch 1-2, burpee , side kick left , burpee, side kick right. Repeat 1 minute.					
Alternating Side Kicks (Left lead and Right) In fight position throw waist level side kick. Pull back and repeat. 50 then switch lead leg.					

19. Your Optional and Extra Workouts

19.1. TRACK Workout

Cardio Plan: Month 1 , 2 and 3

	Set	Set	Set	400 Time
Week 1	6 X 100M	2 X 200M	1 X 400M	
Week 2	4 X 100M	4 X 200M	2 X 100M	**no**
Week 3	6 X 100M	2 X 200M	1 X 400M	
Week 4	8 X 100M	2 X 200M	2 X 100M	**no**
Week 5	4 X 100M	2 X 200M	1 X 400M	
Week 6	6 X 100M	4 X 200M	2 X 400M	**no**
Week 7	6 X 100M	2 X 200M	1 X 400M	
Week 8	8 X 100M	4 X 200M	2 X 100M	**no**
Week 9	6 X 100M	2 X 200M	1 X 400M	
Week 10	4 X 100M	2 X 200M	1 X 400M	
Time Trial	<u>200</u>	<u>400</u>	**BEST=**	

19.2. Year 2 and Beyond

[Click]() [Here]()

19.3. MMA Drills

Martial Arts Agility Drills
Add drills at least once per week to your planned workouts

Perform circuit 3 times non-stop.

Do 4 sets of this, with 1 minute rest between sets

CIRCUIT 1

- Burpees: 30 seconds

- Shuffles*: 30 seconds

- Cross Legged Jumping Jacks**: 30 seconds

- Mountain Climbers***: 30 seconds

Total Duration = 12 minutes.

These are basically a simple "boxer" type of movement where you shuffle the feet back and forth in a quick shuffling.
Feet are approximately two feet apart; movement is nice and quick.

**Like jumping jacks, but with each time the legs meet at midline they cross each other. Alternate crossing in-front position.*

***From a push-up position with butt slightly arched up, climb & jump quickly, bringing knees up to chest and back. .*

CIRCUIT 2

- The Walking Lunges: 30 seconds
- 4 count Bodybuilders: 30 seconds
- Walking "Knee to Elbows":   30 seconds
- Box/Tire Ski-mogul jumps: 30 seconds

Total Duration = 12 minutes.

Punch Out Drill

Example for "Jab-Cross or 1-2":

Punch bag in non-stop fashion for 1 minute. Jab-Cross...Jab-Cross...Jab-Cross.

Throw punches with no pausing what so ever. Strike bag as many times as possible. ....**While maintaining exact and proper form**. No Slop.

Now pick another " 2 count combo " (IE: Side kicks left and right).

Fight skills are just the example here, too. Pick a drill that most relates to YOUR sport. Maybe "High Knees" in place so that your knees hit open palms of the hands? Get creative.

Perform these Punch out drills as follows:

- 1 minute rounds with 1 minute rest between each round.

- 10 separate combinations of "Right - Left" movements for a total of 10 rounds and 10 minutes rest. You choose! These will alter from time to time, as you build upon your skill sets.

To monitor performance levels: count the amount of repetitions performed during the punch out drills individually.

The goal here is to increase the number of repetitions performed with each "Test" (Usually monthly). Perform all of the movements with good form and proper technique.

You will need to learn to maintain your proper form even in the face of extreme fatigue.

Different agility sprints (Distance in yards Direction)
Pick 3 and perform 3 sets of each

1. Backward 10yd, Forward 5 yd, Backward 15 yards

2. Back sprint 10yd, turn left, Forward sprint 15 yards

3. Back sprint 10yd, turn right, Forward sprint 15 yards

4. Zig-zag, diagonal cuts on 45' angles for 30 yards 30

5. 50% speed sprint, fake left, cut right & explode 25 yards

6. 50% speed sprint, fake right, cut left & explode 25 yards

7. 50% speed sprint, fake right, fake left, cut right & explode 25 yards

8. 50% speed sprint, fake left, fake right, cut left & explode 25 yards

9. Backpedal 10 yards, side shuffle right 5 yards, Back sprint 15 yards

10. Backpedal 10 yards, side shuffle left 5 yards, Back sprint 15 yards

12. Crossover right, sprint 10 yards, shuffle 5yards

13. Crossover left, sprint 10 yards, shuffle 5yards

14. 15yards Drop right- Open hip right, drive off left leg, sprint at 45' angle

15. 15yards Drop left- Open hip left, drive off right leg, sprint at 45' angle

16. Forward, side shuffle right, backward, forward sprint 10-5-5-10

17. Forward, side shuffle left, backward, forward sprint 10-5-5- 15

19.4. Body Weight Workouts

Workout "A"

1.) Dead Lift

2.) Barbell Shrugs

3.) Bench Press

4.) Ass-to-Grass / Low Squats

5.) Overhead Barbell press

6.) Dips
   (Since dips ARE your body weight...No weight is prescribed)

7.) Hanging leg raises (No weight)

Workout " B "

1.) Barbell Alternating Lunges (Stationary & Some cheating allowed)

2.) Barbell Bent rows

3.) Barbell Incline Press

4.) Dips (See above at workout A)

5.) Reverse Grip Pull-ups (See Dips)

6.) Barbell Shrugs

7.) Bench Leg raises (No Weight)

20. Support Website , Printable Forms and Supplements Store

CLICK HERE

21. Grocery List

Grocery list for The Program
(Monthly)

Not everything needs to be purchased at one time or every time, however everything on the list should be on-hand in your kitchen.

Complex Carbohydrates & Fibrous Vegetables

Sweet Potatoes
Peas
Carrots
Brown rice
Green beans
3 Pounds of Pasta
1-2 Bag fresh Spinach
Oatmeal
Green peppers
2 Loaf of Whole-grain bread
Cucumber
Yogurt
Broccoli
Squash
Peanut Butter and or Almond Butter

Fruits

10 grapefruits / Lemons or Cans of (Half can per week day)
All-natural Applesauce
Frozen Strawberries
Raisins

Proteins

2% milk
15 chicken breasts
4 dozen eggs
Ground Turkey
Ground beef
Skim Cottage cheese
10 cans Tuna (The perfect "protein Lunch")

Juices (100%natural)

Orange Juice
Apple juice
Cranberry
Grapefruit

Fats

Coconut oil
Canola oil
Olive Oil
Peanut & Almond Butter

Food Supplements once per Month

- <u>Whey protein powders (25 to 30 servings)</u>
- <u>Skim Milk Powder</u>
- <u>Vitamin and Minerals</u>
- <u>Creatine (Alternating with L-Glutamine - below - every other month)</u>
- <u>L-Glutamine</u>
One Case of Ensure Plus or Slim-fast (on-hand for quickies on-the -go)

22. OPEN

23. Glossary

GLOSSARY

Aerobic- Aerobic is anything which increases oxygen consumption by the body. Aerobic exercise is a low intensity longer duration exercise like cycling.

Anaerobic- Anaerobic is reactions which do not require oxygen to occur. Weight lifting although it increases heart rate and breath rate is an anaerobic activity because the muscle tissue has anaerobic metabolisms.

Antioxidants- Compounds at the cellular level which combat free radicals to reduce oxidization of the body tissues.

Barbell – A free weight apparatus consisting of a long bar with plates added to each end for resistance. Used in exercises like barbell Bench Press, Biceps Curls and Squats where two hands are required to hold the bar.

Calories- A unit for measuring the energy provided by foods.

Carbohydrates - Any of a group of organic compounds that includes sugars and starches, celluloses and gums and serves as a major energy source in the diet of all creatures. Carbs Are compounds produced by photosynthetic plants and contain carbon and hydrogen and oxygen.... usually in the ratio 1:2:1

Carbing up – Carbing up is the practice of depleting your body of carbohydrates then systematically loading up again.
The theory is if you exercise and eat the proper types of carbohydrates you can store more than you could originally by tricking the muscle cell in a deprived carbohydrate state.

Cholesterol – A substance found in animal tissues and various foods that is normally produced in the liver and is very important as a constituent of cell membranes and a precursor to steroid hormones. Its level in the bloodstream can influence certain conditions, such as the development of atherosclerotic plaque and coronary artery disease. There are two types of cholesterol: HDL, which is the good cholesterol and LDL, which is the bad Cholesterol.

Compound Exercises - Compound exercises require more than one muscle group to perform. These types of exercises are excellent for building mass and training more muscles in less time.

Cycle – Training phases last one cycle. A cycle determines the length of a training phase. There are three different training cycles depending on your level of fitness. The harder you can train the more advanced of a cycle you follow. The more advanced a cycle the more recuperation time between workouts.

Dumbbell – A free weight made of a short handle consisting of weight plates on each side for resistance. One hand is required to use a dumbbell.

Glycemic Index - The glycemic index is a useful tool that measures how fast a particular food is likely to raise your blood sugar. Pure glycogen has a rating of 100 and raises blood sugar levels very quickly. The lower the number the slower the particular food breaks down. Foods high on the glycemic index are good for post – workout foods to replenish blood sugars rapidly. High glycemic foods are also more likely to be stored as fat. Lower glycemic foods are a better choice throughout the day for sustained energy and less likely to be stored as fat.

Glucose – Glucose is the major source of energy for use by the body. Carbs are metabolized into glucose by your body.
Any excess glucose is converted to glycogen and stored in your liver or fatty acids and stored as fat.

Glycogen- The main form of carbohydrates stored by the body that is readily converted to glucose to supply energy to the muscles.

Hyperthyroidism- Over productivity of the thyroid gland that is producing abnormally high amount of thyroid hormones compared to the accepted average.

Hypothyroidism- An abnormally slow thyroid compared to the average human measured by the amounts of thyroid hormone being produced.

Isolation Exercises – Isolation exercises require only one muscle group to perform. These types of exercises are great for specializing on weak muscles and areas. Examples of isolation exercises are Leg Extensions and Preacher Curls.

Macronutrient – A term for the groups of nutrients that include your proteins, your carbohydrate and your fat.

Micronutrient – A term for the individual vitamins or minerals your body requires .E.g. Vitamin C is a micronutrient.

Oxidation – The act or process of adding oxygen. The addition of oxygen has negative effects to the human body which have shown responsible for degenerative disease.

Phase - Each method of training is called a "training phase". If you are doing drop sets you are in the drop set training "phase". If you are doing rest-pause training you are in the rest-pause training "phase". Each and every phase lasts for exactly one cycle. Then the next type of training phase begins.

Repetition- A repetition is one full cycle of an exercise movement. As an example if you performed 10 repetitions of leg extensions you have completed ten full cycles of raising the weight to completely contract your thighs fully then lowering the weight to the starting position.

Set- A set is a group of repetitions performed together with no break between. For example to perform three sets of 10 repetitions of biceps curls you would perform ten full repetitions of curling the weight from the start position to the fully contracted position then back to the start position again ten times then taking a short break or rest. Repeating the process again two more times to equal three sets.

Standing Heart Rate- Standing heart rate is your hearts beats per minute when you are well rested or have not done any type of movement for a little while. It is your heart rate when you have been sitting around watching a movie or doing no physical activity.

Superset- Two exercise movements performed one after another with as little rest as Possible.

Supinate- This is turning or rotating (the hand or forearm) so that the palm faces up or forward.

Warm up Set(s) - The first set(s) of an exercise performed for a body part solely to warm up the muscle(s) to prepare for injury free intense training. Warm up sets are not for stimulating muscle growth rather just to prevent injury.

Working Set(s) - The last set(s) performed for an exercise after the muscle is thoroughly warmed up. These sets are the ones that are monitored carefully to increase work loads every workout.

Made in the USA
San Bernardino, CA
22 December 2017